Route 47

Molly Faris

Grateful acknowledgement is made to Mary Mann and Ronald Zastre.
Cover art by Coleen Patterson

I dedicate these pages to my family and yours,
All the people who spend their days helping others,
The Gallery,
My Mother,
And to my Father.

The Tribute

"What is up with his lips?" Kate shouts.

I look at Dad lying there. "Wow! That *is* horrible."

Kate places the golf tees in the casket. Mom approaches and cries, "Oh no, it doesn't even look like him. Oh Richard, I can't believe this, it looks nothing like you."

The lady from the funeral home comes in and asks, "How is everything?"

"What's wrong with his lips?" Kate replies.

Mom interrupts, "It looks nothing like him."

She places a scorecard in Dad's pocket. A man carrying a black tackle-box walks in and asks, "What doesn't look right?"

"His lips are all messed up," Kate sighs.

Mom cries, and whispers, "It just doesn't look like him."

"The lips are definitely a problem," I add, "but he looks way younger or something."

"I matched the pictures best I could. If you want, I can fix his lips."

He sets the tackle-box down and asks, "What is wrong with them?"

"The sides never went up like that," Kate replies. "The ends are too high."

"All right, just give me a few minutes, please."

I'm intrigued as he opens his box, but the funeral lady says, "If I could please have you step outside while he works on him."

We follow her out to the foyer to a table with a television. She says, "This is the slide show we made of the pictures you gave us."

She turns and walks back into the chapel.

I stare at the screen, but become enraged, for I want to know what is going on in there.

I have been through every step of dying in complete detail with him, and I can't watch that fuck play around with his lips? Bullshit!

Determined to watch the man fix Dad's lips, I open the chapel door, but the lady blocks my way to the casket. "I'm sorry, he isn't finished yet," she says, putting her arm around me, and leading me back to the television screen.

The realization hits me—*this is the end. It's finally over. He is out of my hands and not my mission anymore.*

"Okay," the funeral lady announces, her head peeking through the chapel door. "We are all set, if you would like to come back in."

I follow Kate and Mom back into the room. The man is closing the tackle-box.

Kate is the first to the crate, "Oh, much better."

I walk up close to the body, but still don't recognize the man lying there. It's a young man, and reminds me of some movie star, no wrinkles, very smooth, and tan. It is distressing to look at a face that does not resemble him. He wore many faces these past few weeks, but this is the last.

"It just doesn't look like him," Mom cries.

"Well, it's like a younger version," Kate replies.

I am overcome with anger, "Whatever! It's just amazing how everything always gets fucked up for us. I mean, he looks like Robert *fucking* Redford, for Christ sake."

"Molly, you are in church. What is wrong with you? You and that word!" Mom shouts.

Jason, the assistant pastor, walks in and embraces Mom, "I'm so sorry, Tweedy."

He turns to me and says, "I'm sorry about your dad. He always made me laugh."

I grin, "Yeah, he was pretty funny."

We stand awkwardly, staring into the casket.

"Molly, there is something I'm curious about. You see, Pastor told me about your dad and the visions he had. He said your dad was reaching out with his arm. I have heard that when people do that, they are reaching for Heaven. I wanted to ask you something about that. He had a tumor under his arm and he could barely move it, right?"

"Yeah, I had to clean it every day and when I lifted his arm he screamed in pain."

"So, when he reached, he did not use that arm, the one with the tumor?"

I think for a moment, drifting back to The Scene in the living room before Dad died.

"Oh my God, Jason, he did it with both arms. He did use it, all the time. When I cleaned it he always got upset. But you're right, when he reached out he lifted it up way high, very high. Wow, that's crazy, how didn't we notice that?"

"That is quite amazing. I guess, when there is complete peace, there is no pain. Your dad is obviously in a wonderful place."

I hear voices outside the chapel and turn around to see Curtis, Christy, and Cody enter the room. Tears fill my eyes as Curtis approaches the casket. He stops at the edge and looks down at Dad.

"Hey, Pops," he says, as his hand glides down Dad's blue blazer. "Good, you got your golf shirt on, and your tees there, and your putter. You're all ready to go, Dad."

He tries to clear his throat, but blubbering comes out instead as he cries out, "I love you Pops. I'm gonna' miss you so much."

Kate sits down in the front row, facing the casket. I join her and we begin a long day of goodbyes.

Mom says, "Aunt Judy is here."

I turn around and I'm reminded of Grandma Betty, Dad's mom. She died when I was very young, and all I remember of her is purple. Her entire house was this color, including the carpets, the walls, furniture, and even the dishes. Her daughter, Aunt Judy, today wears a lavender suit and shoes to match. She is unsteady with her cane as she approaches the coffin holding her little brother.

"Oh, baby bro. Oh, baby bro," Aunt Judy sobs, as she lunges toward his cold, still form.

Kate runs to her and pulls her back. Mom approaches with tears and I get up to huddle with them. The moment I've anticipated is before my eyes—*the body, the casket, and the father, they are one.*

He was a little guy and always wore tinted glasses. I barely ever saw his bright blue eyes, until recently. His forever-wavy, silver hair still glistens on the pillow, and I can't help but stroke it. Panic consumes me. I can barely breathe, and I make an embarrassing snort, "I just love your hair. It was always like this, always."

Tears fall to my cheeks and I whimper loudly. Mom grabs me into her chest, "I know, Molls, I know."

Kate and I now sit, staring at the coffin, as people come in and out. They all approach him in a similar style, hands folded together, hanging low and limp, then stand flat-footed with a bit of a tilt as they examine the corpse.

"Well, well, look who decided to show up," Mom whispers.

Claire struts by without acknowledging us. Not even stopping at the casket, she makes her way to the other side of the chapel where her daughter, Bridgett, is.

Claire is my half-sister; a soul bathed in self-pity and envy for years. She has spent most of her life in a bed of depression. Many doctors tried to help her, but as one put it best: *Claire is the most manipulative, illusive, slippery patient I have ever had.*

My dad, the guy in the box, is Richard, better known as Dick. He married young and had three children: two girls, Kate and Claire, and a boy, Curtis. While he was married he had an affair with Tweedy, who worked for him as a waitress at The Avenue, his bar and restaurant. He divorced his wife and married Tweedy. He was eighteen years older than her. When they had me, he was forty-seven. His other three kids were all grown up, in their twenties, when I was born.

We all stand at the fabricated oak crate. Curtis's wife, Christy, is first at the door as people enter the room. She can barely stand up, practically falling into everyone. As guests approach her, she slurs out, "I'm Dick's daughter-in-law."

My brother Curtis is right behind her, trying to hold her up.

He has been doing this his whole life.

Next in our dysfunctional line is Claire, who is right in front of Kate, but not one word is said between the two sisters. As kids they were inseparable, but they hardly speak anymore.

I stand behind Kate, with Mom behind me, next to the sight they have all come to see. Many people wait in the hall to approach our line, another ritual of this process of death, which I'm living.

Several hours later, Mom and I are finally sitting down, conversing with friends.

The funeral lady comes in and says, "You can stay as long as you like, but the visitation is now over."

"Thank God, we're done," I reply.

Kate runs in and yells, "There's a *forty-seven* in the video."

I turn, "What?"

She grabs my hand, "Come on."

I look at everyone, "You've got to be kidding me. I guess it's not over yet."

Mom follows, as does everyone else. We watch the pictures change on the screen. "We have a while to go because we just saw it," Kate explains.

Chloe, Curtis's daughter says, "It's crazy! I mean, I watched it all day and I never saw it."

"We've seen this a hundred times. Who noticed it?" Mom asks.

"Kate did," Chloe answers.

Mom looks at Kate, "You just noticed this now?"

"Yes, Tweets. Now watch, it should be coming up."

"This is it! There it is, on the bottom," Chloe yells.

"Oh, it's his high school sweater," Mom sighs.

"How didn't we notice that in the actual picture?" I ask.

"I have no idea," Chloe replies. "I picked out that picture and I don't remember seeing the number."

We stand in disbelief and wait for the picture to appear again.

"Oh, there it is," Mom points.

We all lunge toward the screen, staring at the number and the young boy who wore it.

We wait another round to see it again. Mom says,

"Okay, it's the one after this."

Everyone leans in once more, but it's the same result, Dad in a black sweater with the number 47 in white.

Mom, Kate, and I walk back into the chapel after saying goodbye to the final guests. Now it's just the three of us. Mom strokes his head and says, "Goodbye Richard. We will see you tomorrow."

"Bye Dad, I love you," Kate says, as she leans and kisses him.

"Night Dad," I whisper. My hand glides down the silk of the coffin. We leave the room in single file.

I shout out, "See you in the morning, Redford."

Kate laughs.

"Oh Molly," Mom moans.

*

I was up all night, sitting and staring at the spot where the deathbed had been. Finally, I see light peeking around the shutters, and rise to begin this dreaded day. Today is the *fourth* day of the *seventh* month of my thirty-third year of life. Today is my dad's funeral. I have been here for over fifty days, waiting for this to be over.

I just have to get through the eulogy, and I should look presentable reading it.

In the bathroom mirror, I can't believe how big the bags are under my eyes. My face is blotchy and pale. My blue eyes are dim, my blonde hair is dull, and the gray turtleneck doesn't help much. I try to form a smile, but my reflection tells me that this is not a good idea.

I boldly say to the mirror, "I can do this. I'm stronger than most. This is nothing. Piece a cake, Molls, piece a cake."

Those words have echoed before in this room.

About sixteen years ago, in the heat of junior golf, an early morning prepping for a challenging round was common. This mirror was the center of many of my pep talks. Even though it was early, Dad would have already been on the golf course, but not the one I was going to.

The reflection I see today is the same as it was then—fatherless.

*

Next to the casket, Claire and Bridgett stand at his side, as the funeral lady takes off the wreath.

"What are you doing?" Claire asks.

"We are going to start now. I have to close the casket," the funeral lady replies.

"Close the casket?" Claire questions. "Why are we closing the casket?"

"That was the family's wishes."

I get up, walk toward Claire, and ask, "What's going on?"

She snidely answers, "The casket isn't going to be open during the funeral?"

"No."

"But we are not going to get to say goodbye to him."

"Say goodbye to him? You didn't have time to say goodbye to him?" I snap.

"I had hope, unlike everyone else, who wanted him to die. Now, I would like one final goodbye with my father."

"Well, that's why *you* were supposed to be here at ten."

"We weren't here at ten," she whines.

"Well, that's not my problem."

All eyes are on me, as I turn to face the funeral lady, "Can we keep the casket open?"

"I'm sorry, it's already been decided."

"Well, when the funeral is done, can we reopen it and have one last goodbye?"

She tilts her head, "I guess we could do that, for just a

moment though."

"Great, thanks so much," I say.

Claire stands at the other end of the coffin, alone; everyone else is watching and waiting. I turn to her, "Okay, they have to close it for the service, but they are going to reopen it after, and then we can say goodbye to him."

She turns with a devilish eye and huffs, "It's not like it's him lying there anyway. That's not Dad, why would I want to say goodbye to *that*!"

She laughs sarcastically, whips around, and walks to her seat. My hand grabs the casket, tight. I am about ready to scream. I take a deep breath, lean down and kiss Dad's forehead, leaving a lipstick mark. I turn around to walk to my seat. I can't help but smile, seeing my father's friends and family all here; their faces, now wilted, are proof of the passing of time.

Pastor walks by me to the pulpit to begin the service. I sit down. The sermon begins, but I only hear bits and pieces. I am focusing on trying not to blubber. I look down at the paper I am about to read and kiss it, leaving a lipstick mark just like the one I left on Dad. I hear Pastor say my name.

Taking deep breaths, I walk up to the coffin and lay my hand upon it.

I whisper, "Dad, please help me get through this."

My eyes lift up, I see the life-size Jesus on the cross, and I proceed to the pulpit.

I look out at the crowd, and the words roll off my tongue, "My dad was a very funny man. He didn't say much, but when he did, he made you laugh. When you asked him a question, his answer was never predictable and almost always hilarious. He was a stylish man, especially on the golf course. His golf game was similar to his death—slow, detailed, and taken with much thought.

These past weeks became his final round. Many challenging holes and many tough shots…"

My mouth continues, but my mind wanders.

I feel marinated in sadness because this is the distinct end. My father's death was much more than the ending of a life. I watched him linger, as his acceptance grew and mercy healed him. His soul dragged through damnation, but gradually uplifted to what he knew as Heaven.

I was naive to a lot of things until just a few weeks ago, but since then, a wait for death took over my existence. My father's infected body overwhelmed me. He had no physical strength left and even less emotional power, due to his guilty soul. This wait for death turned out to be a game like no other. My mind fades into the past and recalls these fairways of death through life.

The Range

My eyes are trying to open. The phone is ringing, the word 'Mom' is flashing on the screen. It's 6:47 a.m.

"Hello."

Her voice is trembling, "Molly, your dad fell last night and broke his hip. I have been at the hospital all night. He needs to have surgery."

"Is he going to be okay?"

"The doctor says, with his cancer, he is at a high risk, so they are going to monitor him for at least a couple of weeks before they do anything."

"Shit! What's a high risk?"

"I don't know, Molly, but he's not doing well."

"Is he awake? Can I talk to him?"

"Okay. Let me go back in the room. Hold on…Richard, your daughter wants to talk to you."

His breath is deep and raspy. He speaks, "Is that you, Skeeters?"

"Hi Dad, how are you?"

"I'm in bad shape, Skeets."

"I know, Dad, I know. You have to be strong, okay?"

"I will try, Skeets. I will try, but I think I'm losin' the battle."

"Hang in there, you will be fine, I love you, Dad."

"I love you too, Skeets."

His words are soft and weak. He seems worn out from the agonizing world he has been living in. I get the feeling he may not pull through.

Mom's strained voice returns, "Okay Molls, well, I just wanted to call and tell you about your father."

I don't know what to say.

After a moment's pause, she says, "Goodbye, Molly."

I stare at the ceiling, feeling empty. I just moved into this big house by myself, and it's expensive. But money wasn't a problem until just a few days ago, when I was fired from the best paying job I ever had. It was my fault, with thanks to the Christmas party. It hasn't even been a few months since I left my husband.

I seem to fuck up my life at the worst time. It's December 26th. Merry fucking Christmas, Molly.

My eyes are heavy; a tear runs down my cheek.

I remember an easier moment, when I was a kid hitting balls. At the age of eleven, I would walk to the driving range; it was a three-wood away from my house. Dad mowed the grass on the golf course. My favorite time to practice was early in the morning when Dad was working. He always drove up on his mower, the engine was loud and the smell of gasoline strong.

"How ya' hittin' 'em Skeets?"

"Not too bad, Dad. You wanna' see?"

"I gotta' get this done, Skeets, I gotta' tee time later, but I will watch while I mow the putting green. Keep practicin'."

While Dad mowed the range, I chipped and putted on the practice green. Then he would mow the practice green, and I would hit balls down the range.

I find a flight home for the surgery. This will be my first time back since I got divorced. I haven't had much contact with my parents lately. They are not happy with me. I am nervous about how Mom and I will get along with just the two of us in the house. My mom and I never agree on much of anything. I am not about to tell her I lost my job. I will act happy and grateful that they let me take time off.

I'm standing outside O'Hare; it's freezing and slush is everywhere. I'm no longer in Palm Springs, but Chicago, and it's January. The car veers toward me and her face turns to mine. Her cheeks are colorless, her smile is withered.

"How was the flight?" she asks, as I get in the car.

"Fine," I reply.

Her arm reaches out to me, but her face shows disappointment. We clutch each other awkwardly over the center console, for just a second. She pulls out into the stream of airport traffic, and says, "Dad has so many issues including the cancer. He is just getting worse, and it is so draining."

Her hair is blonde and short, but not as neat as usual. Her bright blue eyes have always been sensitive to the sun. She takes off her sunglasses and wipes the corner of her eye with a tissue. She has a few more wrinkles than I remember. I can tell she is exhausted, which is not good, given her heart condition. About six years ago, she had open-heart surgery. I came then, and now, into the same hospital parking lot, straight from the airport, with a parent, to visit a parent.

I follow Mom into Dad's room. He looks horrible. I don't even want to hug him. I barely kiss his lips, and say, "Hi Dad, how do you feel?"

With a harsh crackly voice, he replies, "Like horse-shit."

"That's pretty bad."

"Yeah Skeets, I'm in bad shape."

Mom says, "Well, you have a lot of issues, Richard."

"You don't think I know that, Tweets?"

Mom grabs the television remote. The Golf Channel becomes the center of focus, and nothing more is said.

After a few hours, Mom finally stands up, "I'm tired. I want to go home."

She kisses Dad's cheek, "Richard, we will see you in the morning."

I lean in close to him. My lips graze his neck. I whisper, "Good night, Dad. I love you."

"I love you too, Skeets."

*

It's the next morning, and the glare of the sun off the snow is harsh. We pick up Aunt Judy on the way to the hospital. She is no stranger to this situation. Her husband suffered a stroke that crippled him, and gradually poured out his demise. She has seen a soul endure pain and wither back into its infant-like self. For almost a decade she aided his failing body. His death burdened her more than his illness. It absorbed her to the point of non-existence for too long, and once he was gone, her adaption to everything else became meaningless.

Her husband's death saddened her; however, it didn't soften her up a bit. Aunt Judy has always called a donkey, a donkey. She is the one who will stamp it and deliver it right to your door.

Dad also had a brother, Buck, who died at age forty-one. He immersed himself in alcohol until his drunken gasp let out its final weep. Buck's daughter, Candice, at the age of seventeen saw him first, lying face down on the floor of their living room. She said that her dad was passed out like that all the time, so she didn't think anything of it and went back to her room. But then, a few moments later, she heard her mom scream.

Candice told me that my dad was the first one there at the house, even before the ambulance.

Dad never talked about Buck, but then again, Dad never talked about anything.

Driving to the hospital, Mom says, "He hasn't had radiation on his tumor in over a week, and the nurse says he won't be able to have it until he is recovered from the surgery."

She is crying as she continues, "I can't believe this happened. He was doing so good, just starting to get around again. Now we face another long haul."

It would be best if he didn't make it through the surgery. The lengthy days of despair could end today. It would be difficult, but it would be over, and life would go on, especially for those who need it to.

We arrive at the hospital, and he is already in another room prepping for surgery. We walk in, and he begins to cry, "Hi Tweets."

"Oh Richard, don't cry."

"Don't blame you, Bro. I don't like this place either," Aunt Judy hollers.

"Sis, is that you?"

The surgeon walks in and says to Dad, "Everything looks really good, and in a couple of hours you should have a new hip."

I kiss him, and I know he will be okay, "I love you, Dad."

"I love you too, Skeeters."

They wheel him out of the room, down the hall, and the three of us follow behind, walking with the bed to the elevator. They wheel him in, the elevator closes, and I wonder if it will open again.

As we wait, I think of how much I missed out on the last few years.

I moved to California when I was nineteen. Even at an early age I did not fit in with the Midwestern way. Growing up, the people seemed naive and judgmental of everything. I high-tailed it out West the first chance I got.

Finally, the nurse comes out and says, "He is in recovery right now. He will be moved to room 4-4-7, if you want to meet us there."

Mom says, "Oh, 4-4-7, a new room, this will be his fifth different room since he has been here."

*

Mom and I are driving to the hospital again the next morning. I have to leave this afternoon.

"Mom, I think if he was in California there wouldn't be so much bullshit. Just think if you guys had kept the place in Arizona. Selling that place was the dumbest thing you ever did. Why did you sell it anyway?"

She turns her head, "Oh Molly, get over it, already."

Dr. Howard is in the room when we arrive. Dad is still out of it, but knows we are here. The doctor says, "Richard is the best patient I've ever had. He doesn't say much, but when he does, he makes me laugh,"

All the nurses love Dad too. Everybody loves him. Since I can remember, everyone who meets him thinks he is the greatest guy.

Dr. Howard continues, "I'm sorry to have to tell you this, but he is not strong enough to do the therapy here at the hospital. He can't stay here."

"What do you mean, he can't stay here?" Mom questions, "Where does he go?"

"He will have to go to a nursing home because they have better therapy for him there."

"Oh my God, you're kidding me, a nursing home?" Mom moans.

The doctor reiterates, "The therapy here is too much for him. He can't do it. I will have someone come in to talk to you about nursing homes."

Mom says to me, "I can't believe this."

She turns to Dad, "Dick, do you know what he just said?"

"I have to go to a nursing home."

"That's right. Oh boy, I can't believe this is happening."

"They just tell us he has to leave, and that's it?" I ask Mom.

"Oh yeah, that's how it works."

A nurse walks in and says, "Did you want information on nursing homes?"

"He has to leave here, now?" Mom asks?

"Yes, he needs to be discharged today. "Here's a list of homes, just let me know and I will arrange it all."

"Which one do you suggest?"

"Woodsman East is pretty good."

Mom's voice is immersed in a weeping frustration of heartache, "Oh God, you're kidding me. He was there last year for three months and hated it. He hated it, and you say it's the best one. I can't believe this is happening."

I should stay. This would be the correct thing to do because this nursing home news is devastating. However, I don't want to deal with this, I have to get back and get my shit together.

Mom gets up and puts on her coat. "I'm starving. We are going to go eat before we go to the airport."

I approach him, "Okay Dad, now you get strong and do the therapy."

"I'll try, I love you, Skeeters."

"I love you too, Dad."

I kiss the edge of his lips, and leave the room with an image of his face. I perceive this to be the last vision I will have of him.

We are walking to the car and Mom calls Aunt Judy. Mom is a wreck. Everything in my body is telling me to stay, but I can't bring myself to take the simple steps to modify the circumstance so I can.

The next day he was transferred to the nursing home.

A week later, Mom calls, "Since Dad fell he has not had any cancer treatments. The tumor has spread too much. Molly, he is terminal. The doctor gives him one month."

*

Does this world consist of two souls, good and bad? Good souls become stained, but before their journey on earth ends they are given a chance to be restored to their Heavenly selves. Do confession and forgiveness prove a sinner a good soul?

My father believes in God, but he believes he is not worthy of God. I had no beliefs before these pages. The days to come will conquer my mind, and leave an imprint of a guilty soul's mortality. I stand on the first tee of the most challenging round my father will ever face.

*

Day 1

I arrive in the wee hours of the morning, and my uncle, Mickey, picks me up from the airport. He is my mom's older brother and lives with his wife, Lily, in the city. We will drive out to Mom's in the morning.

I walk in the door behind Mickey, and Buddy, their chocolate lab, greets me. My hands massage his ears and neck, "Hey Buddy, How are ya' doin', boy?"

Mickey whispers, "I guess Lily went to bed. You want something to drink."

"Just water."

I sit down at the antique wooden dining room table, "Hey Micks, do you happen to have any weed?"

"I may have a joint around here somewhere," he hands me a glass of water. "Let me go see what I got."

He disappears into the hallway. When he returns he says, "Sorry Molls, I can't find it."

"No problem, but we will need to stop by Little D's before we go to the nursing home because I'm not going to make it with Mom and Dad, and all this."

"Okay, I'll call him in the morning and tell him we will stop by."

He pauses, then says, "You know, Molls, you and your mom are very strong, it won't be easy, but everything will happen and when it is over you will have gotten through it."

"It just seems so weird because I always thought about my dad dying. He was so much older than my friends' dads. I knew I would be younger than most kids are when their parents die. I just didn't realize it would happen like this, I guess."

"Molls, I don't think anyone ever understands it. When Dixie died, I didn't think I could live without her, but somehow I have. Death has no answers, it just happens, and it sure as hell ain't easy. But you hold onto what you can."

He hesitates for a moment, "It's like when my dad died. Even though I was a kid, I knew he was dead. I climbed from the back seat of the car to his pocket to get a dollar bill before the paramedics got there."

He turns away and walks into the hall. He returns, and sets a dollar bill down in front of me, "See the blood stains?"

I pick up the bill to get a closer look. Mickey explains, "I saw him put that dollar in his pocket. It was change from a hot dog he bought me, and I didn't want them to steal it."

Mickey was only eight when he attended his first Cubs game with his father and uncle. The brothers fought over who was more sober to drive home. My grandfather lost the fight, and then his life.

I let my fingers connect the dark, dirty brown dots on the bill, "Jesus Mick, your dad and Dixie, and what about when you were a medic in Vietnam? Crazy to me."

"I've seen a lot, but Dixie, she was my life."

Mickey's smile and the way his eyes shined when he looked at her always made me curious of love. She was sick for months and had accepted her defeat, but prayed to live to see her daughter get married. As it turned out, Mickey buried Dixie on a Wednesday, and three days later, he walked their daughter down the aisle.

Dad had one suit; it was brown. He only wore it to weddings and funerals, and that week he wore it twice. At the funeral, Dad and I stood closest to Dixie's frame; her hands were neatly folded, and her diamond ring sparkled off her shiny blue dress, the one she was supposed to wear to the wedding.

Mickey went through a rough patch for a few years after her death, but he eventually met Lily and remarried.

*

Mickey, Lily, Buddy, and I set out to the nursing home. They leave for a vacation to Jamaica in a couple of days, and Mom has volunteered to take the dog. It will be good to have Buddy at the house to break the tension.

We make a quick stop at my cousin Little D's house, and I prepare for the days ahead.

We arrive at the nursing home, and walk into Dad's room. Mom says, "There you are. Richard, your daughter's here."

Mom is sitting on the other side of the bed. Curtis's daughter and son-in-law, Chloe and Nate, sit beside Mom. Chloe looks much different from the last time I saw her. She doesn't have her piercings and her tattoos are hidden with long shirtsleeves. She is in her mid-twenties and pretty, with curly black hair tied up in a bushy ball on her head.

I walk right up to the head of the bed, "Hi Dad."

"Hi Skeets."

I lean in to kiss his cheek; an oxygen mask is covering his face.

"Dad, why do you have on that mask?"

He trembles as he holds the mask away from his mouth. "I have…been having problems…breathing."

Lily asks Mom, "Tweedy, what did they say about his breathing?"

"I'm not sure, I haven't talked to anyone. He was like that when I got here."

She changes the subject, "Did Molly tell you she got laid off? I can't believe they laid her off. She got laid off!"

"You did, Molls? What are you gonna' do?" Chloe asks.

Dad's voice crackles, "You think you could get a job teaching golf again?"

I reply, "I'm only going to say this one time—*no more golf*. I'm done!"

Uncle Mickey sighs. My response dims the room.

Dad started me out golfing, but when we actually moved to the course, he became engrossed with his friends. He rarely played with me. In fact, when I was on the high school team he never once stood in my gallery, even though half the matches were on the golf course we lived on. I spent hours on that grass. Those yards of green were my closest friends. I mostly played alone, which is why I never became more than good. Dad was always nearby. He was a wave away: mowing the fairways, golfing with his friends, or sitting on the deck, as I played by. However, a high five after a great putt, he was never close enough to know.

Day 2

We pick up Aunt Judy on the way to the nursing home. We pull up to what I believe will be Dad's death house. My grandma and uncle pull up beside us.

Aunt Judy blurts, "Oh shit, your goofy brother is here."

Uncle Randy is my mom's younger brother. He is not like her, or Mickey, or anyone for that matter. He lives with their mother, hasn't worked in years, and from what I can see, he is missing all of his teeth, except for one lonely crooked fang that leans into his lower lip for support.

Grandma gets out of the car and runs to me. She grabs me with a big smile, "There's Grandma's sweetheart."

I can tell not much has changed; she always looks good and never seems to age. She is eighty-one, but looks like she is sixty-one. Her hair and makeup are always perfect, and her clothes have sparkles and glitters galore.

After her first husband died in the car accident, she remarried the man I knew as Grandpa. He was a disloyal man. Grandma knew of his mistress, but she remained devoted, until the day he died. Then the tides turned, and Grandma had her heyday. Her seventies became her *erotica* years. In fact, for one Christmas, I gave her a deck of sex cards, and the next year, a toy.

We all slide into the room, crowding around the bed.

"How long have you had that mask on, Bro?" Aunt Judy asks.

His hand shakes as he moves the mask up, "Since yesterday, I think, Sis. Hey Molly, can I have some nuts?"

I see them on the table, take the lid off, and hand them to him. He stutters, "Hey Randy, you want some nuts?"

"No thanks, Dick."

"Oh that's right, you can't have any nuts. You have no teeth."

Aunt Judy laughs. I try to hold back a giggle.

Randy is talking and talking about something that doesn't make sense. I want to tell him to shut up.

Aunt Judy glares at him, "Randy, can I ask you a question?"

"Yeah Judy, go ahead."

"Do you ever shut up?"

"I know. I talk a lot."

She shoots back, "Not only do you need to shut up, but you need to get some fucking teeth."

*

As we pull out of the nursing home parking lot, I ask Mom, "Have you talked to Kate?"

"Not since the surgery."

"We need to call her, this is not good."

Kate lives in California, a few hours from me. I call her and tell her that he is on oxygen and can barely talk. I say, "You need to come home because I don't think he will make it 'till the weekend."

Her loud voice is distinctive, "All right, well, I'll look into getting a ticket tonight and let you know."

Day 3

I wake up in the room I grew up in. The walls, the dresser, and the cold frost on the windows haven't changed in twenty years. The smell of the room saddens me. It's too long since I've been here.

Mom goes through a morning routine of watching Golf Channel and fussing around the house. I sit on the couch, waiting for her to be ready. Finally, we head out. On the way to the nursing home, Mom and I are sitting at the stoplight.

Annoyed, I blurt out, "Route 47, fuck, it just doesn't end."

Mom says, "What?"

"Forty-seven. It's everywhere I go. It's just amazing. I don't understand it."

"Oh Molly, you just think about it too much."

I chuckle, "Just wait, you will see how crazy it really is. I'm telling you right now, this number means something. I don't know what it is, but it is everywhere."

"Oh Molly, it's the main road where we live. We go by it every day. Get over it."

"I know, that's exactly the point. Just wait, you will see."

We walk into his room, and Mom yells out, "Oh my God!"

Dad is sitting up in a wheelchair. He looks great. The oxygen mask is gone and he is alert, bright-eyed and bushy-tailed.

Mom says to him in shock, "Richard, you are sitting up!"

"Yeah, I feel a little better today, Tweets."

Mom and I glance at each other with the exact same dumbfounded expression.

I may be here a lot longer than I thought.

"Hey Tweets?"

"What is it, Richard?"

"I think I have to take a shit."

"Now?"

"Yeah, now. Get the nurse."

"Geez and crackers, Richard. Really! Now?"

"Yes, Tweets. Don't be such a donkey nuts. Get the nurse."

"God dammit, Dick. You are unbelievable sometimes."

She gets up and stomps out of the room, and then walks back in with the nurse.

"You want to stay here, or wait in the hall?" the nurse asks.

"Oh, we're okay here," Mom replies.

I agree, "Yeah, we're all right."

I watch, but soon realize, his bare ass-cheeks cupping his elderly testes are not something I want to see.

I could be scarred a long time over this.

Mom turns from the sight, "Why don't we go outside."

Thank God.

The nurse replies, "There is a waiting room just to the left."

Mom and I sit in the waiting room, staring at the television in uncomfortable silence. I can't get it out of my head.

Why would the nurse turn him that way? Did she do that on purpose? I mean, she can't honestly think I wanted to see that.

I finally break the silence.

"I told Kate he was going to die in a few days."

Mom says, "What a difference from yesterday. He is the best he's been through this whole thing. When Kate gets here we will have to explain to her how bad he was yesterday. How were we supposed to know he was going to do a one-eighty?"

Now back in his room, we all stare at the television, mostly in silence. Less than an hour later, Mom says, "Well Dick, we have to get going, we are playing cards at Tracy's today. We will be back later. Do you want us to bring you anything?"

"A shake," he shouts.

"A shake?" I ask.

"Okay, we will be back, I'd say, about five, with your shake," Mom says.

Poor man is dying, and we are going to go play cards. Typical for my family, so I'll go along with it.

*

We pull in our driveway, Mom says, "I'm letting Buddy out, and then we will walk over."

While she is preoccupied with the dog, I run to the downstairs bathroom. I smoke a big, fat bowl of grass, cover myself in body spray, and fly back upstairs.

Mom and I walk into Tracy's house together, and I am struck by the sight of the Midwestern housewives, my parent's neighbors, who are almost all new to me. Growing up, there weren't as many houses in the cul-de-sac.

We are playing a game called *Hand and Foot* that uses a minimum of four decks of cards, depending on how many players there are. Hours have gone by and we just started our second game. Mom is having a blast—she has forgotten about her world momentarily. Her phone rings.

It's bad news.

Her head falls. She croaks, "The hospital? He's going back to the hospital?"

We all sit silent, anticipating the response.

"They are taking him now?" she says.

She pauses, and then shakes her head, "Okay, thank you, goodbye."

She begins to cry as she explains, "They are taking him by ambulance to the hospital because he has pneumonia."

She struggles to continue, rising from the table, she heads down the hall, "We have to go, I'll get our coats."

Someone is talking to me, but I don't hear anything. I don't see anything. I am cemented to the floor. I start to cry, and say, "Oh no, my sister needs to get here. She has to make it."

I run into the bedroom where Mom is, "Come on, we need to go."

She puts her jacket on. She is accustomed to this situation. She is tired. She has been in and out of the hospital and the nursing home too many times with him. She is ready to move on.

In the car on the way, I say to her, "I can't believe this is happening after how good he looked this morning."

Her tone is stricken with despair, "This is the way it is, Molly. It's a frickin' roller coaster. I have been doing this for years."

We now sit in the emergency room, waiting. I hate not knowing what is going to happen. Mom says to me, "Now Molly, I don't want you to get mad at me, but what really happened between you and Trent?"

"Really? You want to do this now?"

"I can't believe that, after the beautiful wedding you had. You were so in love."

"Oh Mom, you and your blinders. We got married on an island, of course it was beautiful. What you see in the picture is not always the truth. It's just a mirage. Almost everything is. Plus, Trent drank a lot, and it really bothered me."

She is surprised, "What? He did?"

I don't respond because it's best to let her ponder it.

An hour later, Mom tries again, "What do you consider drinking a lot?"

"Mom, I'm done with this. I am tired and I don't want to sit here anymore, and I sure don't want to get into this. I hated the way he acted when he drank. I couldn't take it anymore. Now, I don't want to talk about it. I am tired, and I just want to get this over with."

"Well, you never told me any of that."

She is right, I didn't. I didn't tell her much and never have. It's hard to tell her things without feeling judged.

A nurse finally walks us back to the intensive care unit.

"Hi Richard, what happened?" Mom says.

"I don't know. They took some X-rays, and then they rushed me over here. Who won at cards?"

Mom grabs one hand and I grab his other.

"Now, we were not going to tell you, but I think you should know, someone is coming to see you tomorrow. Do you know who it is?" Mom asks.

"No," he says.

"Katie is coming to see you tomorrow."

He begins to cry, "I think it's a good thing you told me."

I choke up and a fart-like sound comes from my nose as I try to hold in my emotions. Mom's phone rings, and she walks out of the room.

I'm standing at the bed, looking at him. His cheeks are a creamy color and his skin is shriveled. Purple veins, defining the lines of age, stand out from his milky forehead, but the silkiness of his thick, wavy gray hair is just like I remember. I look around the room, identifying each item I see. There are all sorts of medical gadgets.

Will all these items be here when he dies?

Dad, all of a sudden says, "So Skeets, I saw this commercial today for a cancer treatment center. They said they treat all kinds of cancer. You need to get the number and give them a call."

I have no idea what to say.

"Oh yeah, well, we will see, Dad. We will see."

My hand rests on his shoulder and my toes scrunch the floor in the effort of supporting my wobbly knees.

He is going to die in this room.

Mom walks back in and says, "Curtis is on his way, and I left Claire a message."

She sits down, "I hope we are not here all night."

"What do you mean?"

"We have to wait 'till he gets in a room. This is intensive care, he needs to get a hospital room."

I know he can hear everything we say even though his eyes are closed. I look at him.

Nope, not this room.

Curtis walks in only minutes later. He walks right up to me and gives me a hug. He practically yells in my ear, "Molly Dee-Dos. How are ya' lil' sis?"

"Oh, I've been better."

His voice softens a little as his arms loosen from my body, "Yeah, I know."

He turns to Dad, "Hey Pops, how ya' holdin' up?"

Dad's voice crackles, "I feel all right, but they rushed me over here."

Curtis looks exactly the same. He has a crazy mustache, long and thick, with the ends going down past the corners of his lips. His brown hair is a bit longer than I recall, but it is full and wavy, just like Dad's.

Curtis's son, Cody, is with him. Cody looks like he should be admitted into the next room. His eyes are worse than blood-shot and his face is covered with sores, or zits, or something.

It's so bizarre to be in this setting. I have always wondered about Dad's death, but always from the periphery.

I watch Curtis stand over the bed.

I feel guilty for moving away and not being a part of my dad's life for very long. Curtis has been with him his whole life. Curtis, Claire, and Kate, his other kids, all worked for him at The Avenue. I was six when he sold it. I don't have half of the memories they have. I haven't been home in three years. Now, I am here only because he is going to die.

Curtis tells Dad to stay strong and fight. He says, "You gotta' hang in there Pops. We aren't ready for you to go yet."

*

Curtis and Cody are gone, but Mom and I are still waiting. It has been almost six hours.

The nurse comes in and says, "They finally got him a room. I'm sorry it took so long, but this was the first room available in almost three hours. It's been a crazy day. Anyway, room 4-4-7 is where he is going. Do you know how to get there?"

Mom says, "Oh yeah, we know how to get there. He was in that same room the last time he was here."

We get up to the room. I walk up to the door and take a picture.

Mom asks, "What are you doing?"

"You don't think it's a bit strange that he is going to die in this room?"

"Come on Molly, I want to get out of here. It's been a long day. Now, say goodnight to your father."

I watch his frail features fade away into a sound rest, "Dad, now you hang in there for Katie. We will see you tomorrow. I love you."

Mom pushes against me and grabs his arm, "Okay Richard, we will see you tomorrow. Katie will be here."

She leans into his cheek and kisses him. I walk to the door, again examining the number on it. Mom hurries past me, "Come on Molls, I want to get out of here."

Finally, back at the house, I lie in bed, but can't sleep. I stare at my hands, wanting to put them together, but scared to admit it. My fingers finally interlock and I pray, "Dear God, let him live a couple more days so he can see Kate. Please Lord, it's really important that she sees him."

Day 4

I wake up and walk out to the living room. Mom is sitting in her recliner reading a book. Before I know it, a couple hours have gone by.

I finally say, "When are we going to go?"

"We will go get Kate first and then go to the hospital."

I figured we would go to the hospital first, but I can tell she is fed up with everything. I have only been doing this for a few days, and I am emotionally drained. Mom has been doing this for weeks, months, well actually, years. I can't even imagine how she did this when she was still working. We live out in the country, forty miles from the hospital, and it's the middle of the winter. If she wants to wait and go later, that's fine by me.

*

We circle the airport for the sixth time, and I hope, it is the last, since I am scared for my life. Mom drives like a maniac; there are people and cars all over the place, and nobody is paying attention to anything.

I spot a tall woman with full, curly brown hair to her shoulders.

"Is that her? What is she wearing?"

"Well, Molly, she hasn't been here in years, she

probably doesn't have many winter clothes."

"Obviously, since it looks like Bill Cosby gave her that sweater."

Kate gets in and we head straight to the hospital. Mom spends the hour-long car ride telling Kate everything she has been through with Dad over the last month.

When we get to his room, he has his shirt off, and there are nurses everywhere.

"What is going on?" Mom asks.

A nurse turns around and says, "He became very hot. We are trying to cool him down."

Mom pulls Kate through the nurses, "Richard, look who's here."

"Hi Dad, how are you feeling?" Kate asks.

"Katie, I'm not doing too well."

"I know Dad."

As if on cue, Curtis walks in with Chloe. Ignoring the commotion, he yells, "Hey Pops, how ya' feelin'?"

Curtis notices Kate, and his arms go out to her, "Katie, hey Sis!"

We all greet with hugs.

It is so strange to be together in this hospital room.

Dad says, "My feet are on fire! Please, rub my feet."

Mom starts to rub his feet, and he moans, "That feels so good, Tweets. They are burning up."

He is in constant pain. Once again, he commands, "Can you guys please move me. My crack is killing me. Maybe you can put a pillow under it."

"Okay Gramps, we can try that," Chloe says. "Come on Dad, you lift him."

Curtis lifts his hips a little bit, and Chloe and I try to shove the pillow under him.

"Oh, that won't work!" Dad screams as Curtis tries to

position him. "Molly, call the nurse, maybe she can make me more comfortable."

"Dad, you can't keep calling them in here just to reposition you."

"But Molly, I'm in so much pain, my crack hurts so bad."

A lady in scrubs, carrying a clipboard, comes in and says, "You need to set up an appointment with hospice."

She hands Mom a folder containing information on the hospital's hospice.

Curtis says, "Claire needs to be here when we talk to hospice."

Mom says to the nurse, "Let me try to get a hold of his other daughter."

She opens her purse and fumbles inside it, looking for her phone. She finally finds it in her coat pocket.

"Hey Claire, it's Tweets," she says into the phone. "We need to schedule a meeting with hospice for your father, and I need you to call me back as soon as possible."

After a few hours, we are walking to the car, and Mom says, "I thought Claire would have called back by now."

"Yeah right, she won't call back tonight. That's Claire, always on her terms," Kate snickers.

*

Due to the fact Kate is here, I lost my bed. I could sleep downstairs, but I think I would be too scared, so I decide to sleep in the living room. There is this doorbell light shadowing the room. It looks like something that would be in a funeral home, a square box with wood trim and stained-glass that light shines through. It's eerie. I noticed it the day we moved into this house.

Mom was not too excited about this particular house, but Dad loved it. He had just gotten the job mowing the golf course and this house sat perfectly on the 2nd hole.

Day 5

Mom and Kate are in the kitchen. Mom notices me waking up, and says, "Molly, we are going to be leaving soon, you need to get ready."

On our way out the door, my eye catches a check on the counter. It wasn't the check I noticed, but the number of the check. I say, "Oh man."

Mom says, "What now?"

"Did you know this was number 1047?"

"Oh Molly, you are going to drive me nuts."

"Well it is."

"It is? Let me see it," she grabs it. "Oh God, it is."

"That's how it is. You'll see."

Kate asks, "What the hell are you guys talking about?"

On the way to the hospital, I tell her of my mysterious number.

We walk in his room and I can immediately tell he is much better today. "Hi Skeeters."

Kate and Mom small talk for a while, until Dad says,

"When do I get to go home?"

We don't respond.

He loudly asks again, "Hey Ma, when am I going home?"

Mom answers, "I don't know Dick, I don't know if you are coming home."

"Did you get the prescription for my scooter?"

"We are not going to get a scooter."

"Well, how am I supposed to get around? I have to sit at the table to eat! How am I going to sit at the table?"

"Richard, you're not going to sit at the table. You can't get out of the bed."

Claire's daughter, Bridgett walks in, bursting, "Oh my God, Aunt Kate, I didn't know you were coming."

Kate stands up, and they embrace.

Bridgett works in the maternity ward downstairs. She has long blonde hair. She looks a lot like her mother but, fortunately, does not have her mother's internal qualities.

She walks close to the bed, "Hi Gramps, how are you feeling?"

"Better than yesterday. I am ready to go home."

Mom interrupts, "Bridgett, have you talked to your mother?"

"I did yesterday."

"Well, I called and left her a message. We have to meet with hospice, and she has not called me back."

"Hospice is great. We did it for Blake's grandpa. Yeah, my mom will definitely want to be there."

"Maybe you want to call her then, because we can't be

waiting around much longer. I mean, we are waiting on her as it is."

"All right, I will make sure she calls you tonight."

She leans in to Dad and says, "Gramps, I have to get back to work. I'll be back later to check on you."

As Bridgett walks out, Pastor walks in and hugs me, saying, "Hi Molly, you're home. That's good."

Mom says, "Pastor, this is Dick's oldest daughter Kate, she lives in California too."

They shake hands, as Pastor says, "This is great, Dick. Your family is here."

Pastor hasn't aged a bit, he has put on a little weight, but in a good way, because he was always too thin. He is tall, upright, with long arms and long legs. He used to have a little hair on the sides, but it's all gone now. He is dressed in slacks and a black winter jacket.

I saw a lot of Pastor when I was young. I went to a private Lutheran school that is attached to his church. Most grade school days he was in my sight, but I never imagined he would be so visible today.

Pastor asks, "Would you like to take a communion together?"

Dad replies, "Yes."

Pastor opens a little wooden box containing all he needs. He pours the wine from a little decanter into tiny cups and hands each of us one.

I don't want to drink the wine. This situation is pissing me off. I do not understand God. I wonder if He is even real. I can't grasp the thought of building something, and then letting it get destroyed. This world is filled with such despair, and I don't see the need. I would think a creator would want more protection of his masterpiece. If God made it, then why can't God fix it?

Don't even get me started on the Bible. Maybe I will write a book of crazy stories and instructions. I will bury it, and hope that in 3,500 years someone finds it and its words become the way of the land. If history repeats itself, then I should start writing.

I put the wafer on my tongue and shoot the wine.

Pastor grabs Dad's hand and says, "Okay, let's pray."

He turns, and with his other hand takes Mom's hand, Mom grabs Kate's hand, who, in turn, grabs mine. I walk closer to Dad, stick my arm over the side of the bed, and clutch his free hand; it is paper thin.

Pastor's words take over, "Lord, we ask you to guide Richard and his family in this time of need. Give us the strength to understand your almighty plan. Thank you for bringing Kate and Molly home. Allow us all the courage to help Richard release his soul back to you, Lord. Amen."

Amen, rolls off my tongue as though I'm used to praying. Our circle breaks and I turn and walk out of the room. I am trying to hold back tears, but just can't. It is too much to take in. I take a few deep breaths.

I step back into the room as Pastor says, "Okay Dick, today is Ash Wednesday. I have to go give a service tonight."

He says goodbye to all of us and makes his exit.

Only a few minutes later, I see Curtis and Cody walking down the hall.

Curtis walks in, shrieking, "Hi Pops, how you feelin' today?"

Dad says, "I feel a little better, but my feet are on fire."

I don't have a lot of Dad memories from the Avenue, but I do recall when Curtis would deliver the beer. He has always driven a beer truck and is wearing the same uniform today: blue pants and a sturdy white shirt with thin blue stripes. It has a pocket with pens on one side and a name patch on the other. His hands are in his jacket pockets. It is a short, navy blue jacket, which also shows his name. He wears light brown work boots tied up at the ankle. His stance is wide, and he sways from foot to foot, while he talks to Kate.

Chloe shows up and we all sit around and stare off into space.

Dad says, "Hey Curtis, I have an idea."

"You do? What's that Pops?"

"You know those dollies you have to haul the beer around?"

"Yeah."

"We could get one of those, you could put me on it, and then wheel me around. You could use the dolly to move me from the bed to the table, and I can eat dinner. I could go home, live another six months, and enjoy my family."

"Boy, you've been figuring this out, but I just don't know if it would work, Pops."

"But, it would be easy."

I ask, "How are we going to get you out of the bed and onto the dolly? You don't have the strength, Dad."

"Well, what do I need to do to get strength?"

"You need to eat."

"I hate this food. It's horrible."

"You have to eat it whether you like it or not. At this time, it is the only thing you can do. Once you eat and get more strength, then we can go from there."

We are in the hallway, and Mom says to Curtis, "I have to schedule this hospice meeting. I can't wait for your sister much longer."

Curtis replies, "Let me try to call her."

Chloe asks, "So Molly, what's up with forty-seven?"

I reply, "I don't know, it's just always around me."

"It is strange, he was in that room when you were here before and now he is in it again. Maybe he knows what it means, did you ask him?"

"Oh shit, I never thought to ask him."

I sprint into his room with Chloe behind me. I grab his hand and say, "Dad, I have to ask you something."

"Okay, Skeeters."

"Do you know what the number forty-seven means?"

"Yeah, that's the year I graduated."

I dart back out of the room and call to Kate in the hall, "Oh my God, Dad graduated in 1947."

Kate yells, "What?"

"Mom, did he really? How don't you know that?" I ask.

She pauses before she says, "Yeah, he did graduate in 1947."

Kate says, "And you were born in 1947, Tweets?"

"Yes, I was born the same year he graduated, 1947."

*

After about five hours, Dad says, "I'm tired now. I'm ready to go to sleep."

We get up and head out, without any hesitation.

We are standing in the elevator, I say, "How about his dolly plan?"

Curtis says, "Dad's a fighter. He isn't giving up that easy."

When we get in the car I say to Mom and Kate, "A fighter? Dad never fought for anything. He was a wimp – fighter, my ass."

Mom and Kate laugh, and the stage opens for a night of, *Dad in Review*.

We have been talking for hours, first in the car and now in the living room, about Dad and the great life he had. I can't believe the things I am hearing. I knew he had it good, but I never really knew *how good* until now.

Mom tells us how they met.

"When I worked at the Avenue I was dating one of the bartenders. One day I got a call at home, and when I picked up the phone, the first thing the guy said was, 'Do you know who this is?' I knew by his voice it was your father."

Kate replies, "Yeah, Dad does have that kind of voice."

Mom continues, "He asked me to meet him for a drink. I said, 'No. You are married.' He told me that he and his wife didn't really have a marriage. He called me every day for a month. I finally agreed to meet him, but I took a friend. We were sitting at the bar, and I asked him, 'So, why are you sitting here with me and not at home with your wife?' My friend elbowed me so hard, I fell off the barstool."

Mom laughs, "I mean, she really knocked me off the barstool. Anyway, he was really nice, and I broke up with the bartender guy, and started to date your dad. We always met outside of town."

She pauses in thought, shakes her head and continues, "Your dad was a ladies man."

Kate replies, "Yes, he was. He cheated on my mom all the time. Tweets, you were not the first."

Mom responds, "Oh, I know, he had another woman while he dated me."

I reply, "What? And you still married him?"

She begins the story, "One day I'm at work at the bank and this big linebacker of a woman comes up and asks for Tweedy. I walk up to her and say, 'I'm Tweedy.' The woman says, 'Stay away from my boyfriend, or I will kick your ass.' I seriously had no idea who she was talking about and asked her, 'Who is your boyfriend?' She screamed real loudly and it echoed throughout the whole bank, 'Dick Weasley!'"

Mom's face fills with anger. She pauses, but soon smiles, "I still didn't learn, because then there was Lulu La Dude."

Kate shouts, "Lulu La Douche! That's what we called her. I remember her, she worked with us at The Avenue. Dad was with her?"

"Oh yeah, I caught them downstairs in the banquet room. They were kissing and all over each other."

"Wow, he probably slept with a lot of employees," Kate comments.

"Oh, I'm sure. I'm telling you girls, your dad was a ladies man."

I reply, "I can't believe it. Dad?"

Kate says, "I believe it, he was always like that."

Mom continues as though she had not been interrupted, "And there was one other one, that I know of."

I reply, "Another one?"

"Oh yes, your father did what he wanted. Let me tell you, he had a very good life."

She explains, "Now, I never told anyone this, but the reason we sold the condo in Arizona was not entirely because of tax purposes. It was because your father couldn't keep his pecker in his pants. He went there by himself, a lot, and it never even fazed me. One day while we were down there, I was sitting at the pool. Molly was swimming and your dad was golfing. A lady sat next to me and told me that your father had taken her out several times. They were dating the last time he was there. I was so mad; I told him either he sells it or he signs divorce papers."

I feel like I'm going to throw up. *I have loathed Mom for years for selling the condo. Dad always told me it was Mom's decision. She protected him, and then I despised her for so much. Now I find out that he was the actual cause. She loved that place. We all did.*

Mom says, "Yeah, he loved his women, but you know what else he loved?"

"His beer?" I reply.

Mom laughs, "Yep, he loved his beer. He was always drunk, and I hated it. God, I hated it."

Kate says, "He was like that when I was growing up too."

Mom says, "He never drank when he was behind the bar, but as soon as he was done working, he was drinking, and by the time he got home, he was drunk."

She pauses, sighs, and shouts out, "And when we moved out here, he did the same thing at the clubhouse!

He would sit up there for hours and get shit-faced with his old cronies after he played golf all day. Oh, he was an asshole."

Kate jumps in to tell a story, "We were all young kids, like nine, seven maybe, and we were leaving The Avenue. Dad and my mom both had a car and Dad was drunk, but he was the one driving us kids home. I snuck in the back seat of her car because I knew Dad had been drinking and I was scared to go with him. I waited for her to get in the house, and then rang the doorbell. I told her that I hid in her car because he was drinking. On the way home, he crashed into a curb and up onto a sidewalk. They all had to go to the emergency room. Claire lost her two front teeth, and Curtis had to have stitches in his forehead and he broke his arm."

Mom interrupts, "I never knew that story."

Kate continues, "He never even got into trouble for it. Everyone knew Dad. The cop that found him was a regular at the bar. Cops came into The Avenue all the time—we all got out of speeding tickets at one time or another."

"What? That's crazy," I say. "No wonder he was the way he was. He got away with everything."

Kate responds, "Well, it did scare him a little, because Dad swore he would never drink again."

"How long 'till he started up again?" I ask.

"Oh, I don't know, a couple weeks."

Kate continues, "I was always surprised, that after what they went through with Buck that Dad drank as much as he did."

Mom replies, "He owned a bar."

"Yeah, first sign," Kate snickers. "You know, one of the

times Buck went to rehab, Dad took him."

"Really, what happened?" I ask.

"Well, he took Curtis, who was only eight years old at the time. My mom was pissed. I will never forget when they got home, and Curtis ran into my room. He was devastated. He said two big scary guys in white had to come out to carry Buck from the car. He said Buck was screaming and fighting them the whole way in."

I ask, "Mom, did you tell me that before?"

"No, I never knew that. Dad never talked. You know how he was."

"Man, I feel like I remember something similar happening, but I don't know."

Kate continues, "Dad actually took Curtis out of school that day."

Mom replies, "You're kidding me, because he didn't want to deal with it. Sounds like your father."

Dad hated confrontation. Curtis was his security blanket for the ride. Most people would not want a child around for such an event. Instead of talking to his brother and giving him hope and strength, Dad takes a distraction to prevent any type of communication.

Kate's voice softens, "What I never understood was, why they continued to let Buck bartend at the bar. I mean, even after rehab he still worked as a bartender. In fact, after one rehab they drove him straight to The Avenue to start working."

I reply, "What? That's crazy. Were they that stupid?"

Kate says, "They were all drinkers. I don't think they understood what an alcoholic truly was."

We sit silent in a moment of Dad's disgrace.

I finally say, "I always thought Dad was hilarious when he drank. Growing up, I actually liked it when he came home buzzed."

Mom shouts, "Hilarious? He was a jerk. In fact, I'll tell you a story that isn't funny at all."

Kate replies, "More? There's more?"

"Your father was a piece of work. Let me tell you, I put up with a lot of crap. He was very upset when I got pregnant. He told me he was too old to have a baby and everyone would look at him funny. He wanted me to have an abortion. The closer we got, the less he had to do with any baby stuff."

I recall Mom telling this before. But the words she breathes next have never been heard, and the picture they leave is frightening.

She begins her story, "I will never forget one night when I was in the kitchen making dinner. I was huge, could barely move. He came home from work, drunk as a skunk. He grabbed a knife and put it on my belly. He screamed at me, 'Tell me I shouldn't just get rid of this baby right now.'"

Kate yells out, "Oh my God! What happened?"

"That was it. He didn't hurt me, but he was a real jerk and he did not want a baby."

Kate says, "I would have been gone and never back."

"What an asshole! I always had my issues with him, but I never knew he was that bad," I yell.

Mom says, "I was the one who did everything. It was my money that got us what we needed. He never spent a dime. When Molly wanted to move to California, he told me that if I paid he didn't care what she did."

She pauses, then continues, "He always made me feel

guilty for spending time with you. He would say to me, 'I'm old and you don't have much time left with me. You will have many years with Molly after I'm dead and gone.'"

This explains a lot, his time was running out and, obviously, was way too valuable for a child. He had already lived that life.

Mom and Kate continue going off about Dad and his ways. Their voices are piercing.

I can't listen anymore. I am deciding if I want to store this information or try to erase it immediately.

I hear Kate say, "And he didn't even buy her a headstone."

I pipe up, "Who? What are you talking about?"

Mom says to me, "Do you know you had another sister?"

"What? What the fuck is going on here?"

Kate says, "You find out a lot of things when people die."

"What was her name?" I ask.

"Christina."

"Of course it was."

Kate says, "I was sixteen. She only lived a few days. We buried her in the cemetery, but Dad refused to get her a headstone. You know what he was thinking: she wasn't worth it. Now it may sound awful, but that's how Dad was."

Mom says, "Do you know what we did the night we got married?"

I respond, "What?"

Mom looks at Kate, "Do you remember, Kate?"

Kate thinks, but can't recall, so Mom says, "We babysat your kids."

Kate yells out, "That's right, you did!"

"We sure did, we had them 'till the next morning."

I laugh, "Is there anything else?"

Mom says, "If there is, I don't know about it."

I look at the clock and scream, "It's 2:47."

"No, it's not that late, is it?" Mom shouts.

Kate gets up and stretches, "Yes it is, we have to go to bed."

I turn the television on because I can't sleep. I can't stop thinking about Mom and all the bullshit she has gone through.

My father needs to let go, so my mother can live her life. I love Dad, but only because he is my father. I came here to say goodbye.

Day 6

I awaken to Mom and Kate's voices continuing from where they left off last night. Mom says, "I always wanted to find him, but your dad refused it."

Mom is talking about her son, whom she gave up for adoption when she was young. I remember when Mom told me; I was about sixteen. We watched a movie about a mother searching for her son. She bawled like a baby through the whole thing, and I could not understand why. She then told me she had a son and she gave him away when he was born.

I never even bothered to ask her what happened. How can I know someone my whole life and not even know something so important?

Kate asks, "How old were you when you had the baby?"

Mom answers, "I was twenty-two."

I rise up, "Twenty-two? Why did you give it up if you were that old?"

"I had no choice. I lived at home with my mom and step-dad. My step-dad would not allow me to bring him home."

Kate asks, "What about the father?"

"The father of the baby was around, but he didn't have any money and couldn't help."

I say, "I don't understand, I mean, you could have done something."

"Molly, what was I going to do? I had nowhere to live. Grandpa would not allow the baby in the house."

Kate asks, "Well, what about your mom?"

"I tried to talk to my mom and convince her to let me keep him."

Kate replies, "That had to be awful."

"It was. The nurses felt so bad for me because all I did was cry."

Kate replies, "What an asshole. I cannot imagine not having a choice in keeping my own baby."

Mom laughs with anger, "He was a jerk. Yeah, my step-dad was a real asshole."

Kate responds, "Yeah, and then you want to find your son and another asshole, my father, forbids you again. You need to find him now."

Mom's voice softens, "I want to."

*

On the way to the hospital Kate says, "Claire will disagree with everything we want to do."

Mom laughs, "Really, ya' think so?"

Claire finally called Mom back last night and agreed to come to the hospital to meet with hospice.

We walk into his room, and Mom with a stern voice asks, "Richard, do you remember Lulu La Dude?"

Kate and I giggle, but there is no reply.

"Richard, do you hear me?"

"Yes, Tweets. Now when do I get to go home?"

"I don't know Richard. We are going to meet with the hospice right now."

She turns to the door, "Come on girls, let's go."

We are headed down the hall to a conference room, where the hospice lady told us to meet her. Curtis is walking toward us and we enter the room together. The woman is already there, waiting for us. We sit down around the big table.

Claire is late, as she always is. I get up and go in the hall to look for her. The elevator doors open, and she steps out robotically. Her head turns looking for direction.

I yell, "Claire, over here."

We make eye contact, but she doesn't move.

"Claire, come on, we are waiting."

Her long, blondish-gray hair sways behind her as she struts over.

She snips, "Are you going to stay out here and make sure no one comes in?"

I reply, "No, *we* are having the meeting."

She growls back, "You are in the meeting?"

With a sarcastic laugh, she enters the room.

The lady describes hospice, and it is not exactly what we thought. If we bring him home we have to take care of him, or hire someone. With hospice, a nurse only comes once every few days, for an hour. We are on our own the rest of the time.

He is completely bedridden. He can't even get out of the bed to sit in a chair. How are we going to take care of him? I see what the nurses do when they come in. What about his tumor? Who is going to do that? I have watched the nurse dress and clean it. We can't do that.

"Well, he needs 24-hour care, how do we get that?" I say.

"Hospice doesn't normally have it. You would have to hire out home care."

I question, "How can't they have that?"

The lady explains, "Hospice is all about comfort, quality of life. We would make it very comfortable for him and you. Once we get him situated, you will be fine. He will come home with all his meds, and gradually he will be taken off of them. He will die in the house. He will not come back to the hospital again."

Claire says, "So we are giving up? Is that what we are doing?"

Mom replies, "The doctors say this is the best thing to do."

"Just to let him die, that's the best thing to do?"

I jump in, "Okay, we have to make a decision."

I look at the hospice lady and sincerely ask, "What do you recommend in our situation?"

"I really can't answer that question. You have to decide, as a family, what is best."

She leaves, and the five of us are left sitting around the table.

Kate says, "I like the idea of home hospice, but I didn't care for that one. Do you know of any others, Tweets?"

Mom shakes her head, "No, but I didn't like that lady either. I would like to talk to someone else. My friend Leslie's husband was at home with hospice, and she said they were great. Let me call her right now."

While Mom is on the phone, Claire says, "What about Dad? He isn't even here, doesn't he get a vote?"

No one answers her. We do listen to her moan and sigh, until Mom hangs up and says, "She said they were great, and she is a paramedic, training to be a nurse, and said she would help us."

"That sounds great," Curtis agrees.

Kate gets up, "Okay, let's go talk to Dad."

Claire marches out ahead of us. Mom, Kate, Curtis, and I walk behind her down the sterile hallway in silence.

I stare at the white tiles of the floor. We approach his door, having no idea what to expect.

Mom, the first in the room, goes straight to the bed. She asks him, "Richard, do you understand what is going on?"

"I know. I'm not getting any better."

"We just had a meeting with hospice. Do you know what hospice is?"

"Yeah. Do I get to go home?"

"Yes, you get to come home."

Claire interrupts, "Dad, do you understand what it means if you go home? You won't be back. That's it."

"I understand. I'm sick and I want to be home with my family and eat Mom's cooking."

Mom says, "I'm going to call them and schedule a time for tomorrow. Now Richard, are you sure this is what you want to do?"

"Tweets, I want to go home, please take me home."

A few minutes later I am standing next to him, feeding him ice chips. My fingers press the ice to his lips. My eyes examine all of us kids.

I'm the one next to him. Everyone else stands in the gallery. Being within the ropes is a different level. It is work to know every shot, and the difficulty of each execution.

Mom says, "We are going to go now, I need to eat something. Outback sounds good."

Dad cries, "Outback! It's too expensive."

Day 7

I wake up from an actual sleep. I wasn't even scared of the doorbell light, but that's because Buddy was with me all night. I stand up and stretch my tangled muscles. This emotional disaster has taken over my body.

On the way to the hospital, I want to tell Mom and Kate that bringing Dad home is a bad idea.

I don't see how this is going to work without a nurse. I mean, who is going to do it all? I know the answer, trust me, I know.

We walk in the room and he eagerly says, "Finally, let's go home. I'm ready."

Mom replies, "Not yet Richard, we are waiting to meet another hospice."

"Why can't I go home now? Why can't you take me home, Tweets?"

Leslie, Mom's friend, walks in the room.

Mom immediately gets up and says, "Leslie! Richard, look who's here?"

Leslie turns toward Dad and says, "Hi Dick, how are you feeling?"

Dad replies, "I'm not doing too well, Leslie. Tweets won't let me go home."

"I'm sorry you are not feeling well, but right now Tweedy is waiting to talk to hospice. Mel was in the same hospice and they were very helpful. They make you very comfortable."

Dad's eyes get real big, "Do I get to go home?"

Leslie tilts her head and smiles, "Yes, you do. You will be home soon."

Doctor Howard comes in; I am happy to see him.

He says to Dad, "How is my favorite patient today?"

"I would be better if I was home."

"Your family is looking into it for you."

I leave the room, and wait for Dr. Howard in the hall. When he comes out I ask him, "What is going on? What should we do?"

He says, "Well, to be honest, it's amazing how the pneumonia is clearing up. It should have taken him within a few days. He's not ready yet, but due to all his other complications, I give him a couple more weeks. Take him home, give him his favorite meals, bring his family around, and he may just make it 'till spring. It would be great if he could see the warm weather. If you take him home he may just make it till then."

Tears form in his eyes and mine as well. He is a doctor, he sees this all the time, and I am surprised he is so compassionate toward Dad.

But spring is a long time away.

Day 8

A short, plump, young woman with black curls tied up in a ponytail is coming toward me down the hall. Her pale skin reminds me of why I left the cold.

I walk back into the room, "This must be her coming now."

She enters and says, "Hi, I'm Courtney from Angel Hospice."

Mom introduces herself, Kate, and me.

Courtney looks at Dad and says, "And you must be Richard."

"That's me. So, how much is this going to cost?"

"Nothing, everything is covered under Medicare."

"I like you, you're hired."

Mom says, "Unbelievable! In your condition how can you be worried about money?"

He replies, "I just want to go home. When do I get to go home?"

Courtney is explaining, and I'm listening to the details.

Mom's health can't be at risk anymore. She needs to keep calm and quiet during all this. I have to take charge.

Courtney continues, "We supply the hospital bed,

oxygen machine, and all the other medical supplies necessary."

I ask, "What about his tumor?"

"The nurse will show you how to do it and everything else he needs done. The nurse assigned to you will be at the house when he arrives. She will have all his information for you, his medication schedule, any dressings he may need changed. You can call us twenty-four hours if any problems arise, and if needed we will come out. Actually, I will come out; I will be your on-call nurse. We could have him home by Monday."

My head is spinning. Shit, that's the day after tomorrow.

Mom says, "What do you think, Pa?"

"Sounds good to me."

We are driving home when I finally speak up, "I think we are screwed. There is no way we can do this on our own."

Mom replies, "We will just have to see, and if we have to hire home care we will. He wants to come home. I have to do what he wants."

I am about to lose my mind. I need a rip of the reefer bad. Mom and Kate continue talking. I'm trying to drown out their voices. I hear Mom say something about my cousin, Little D.

"What is wrong with Little D?" I ask.

"I'm pretty sure he does drugs."

"Oh Mom, seriously. What kind of drugs do you think he does?"

"I don't know Molly, I'm just pretty sure he does."

I reply, "Well until you know more you shouldn't judge."

My anger is rising, and before I know it, I say, "You want to know what he does? He smokes weed."

"How do you know that? You act like you smoke it

too."

"I do, all the time."

Kate lets out a big moan.

Mom starts screaming, "You are my daughter. Oh my God. I didn't raise you like this. What is wrong with you?"

"Mom, it is not a big deal, calm down. Fuck, calm down."

"You curse, you do drugs. Where did I go wrong?"

Kate shouts, "Stop it, stop it, right now! Now Tweets, listen to me. It's legal in California. It's not bad, it's used for medicinal purposes."

"Yeah, it would be great for Dad," I taunt.

"Oh Molly, why did I ever let you go to California?"

"Oh Tweets, don't be ridiculous," Kate chuckles.

Mom doesn't say anything more.

As soon as we get home I go downstairs to the bathroom and absorb a moment of peace. I barely get upstairs and Mom says, "Oh my God, you were smokin' it the day you got here."

I laugh, "What?"

"That's what that awful smell was."

"What smell? Whatever, Mom. You and your Midwest mentality."

"Did you see Little D before you came to the nursing home? I am going to kill my brother. I knew you smelled like smoke. You had this terrible odor to you. It's disgusting. Why do you do that?"

"Do you use vinegar?" I reply.

"Yes."

"Well that has a terrible smell, why do you use that?"

Kate says, "All right, that's enough. Get over it, Tweets."

She looks at her phone, "I just got a text, the kids are

coming tomorrow, they're meeting us at the hospital."

She is referring to her two oldest, who live about 100 miles away.

Mom says, "I'll make a casserole for all of us for dinner tomorrow."

Day 9

"I am so glad we only have one more day of this drive," Mom says.

"Isn't that the truth," I reply, as we pull up to the light at Route 47. "I am so sick of seeing that damn sign."

I launch into a story, "One time when Trent and I were here I almost had him convinced, at like, two in the morning one night, to come here and steal that sign. We were drunk, and I wanted it so bad. He chickened out in the end."

Kate laughs.

"He was just like Dad, a wimp."

"Well, your dad is a wimp," Mom hollers.

We enter his room as his lunch tray arrives. I try to feed him, but he doesn't want it.

"Molly, will you rub my feet?"

On command, I lean down to rub his feet.

I look at him lying there.

I don't want to take care of him at all. He was an alcoholic who was a jerk to my mother, had numerous affairs with other women, never spent a dime on anyone but himself, yet still always managed to get what he wanted. I'm no fucking nurse. He never took care of me, so why should I take care of him? He didn't even want me.

Kate's kids, Tyler and Samantha, come into the room. Tyler is wearing baggy jeans and has a chain hanging from his pocket.

He yells, "Mom!" and runs to hug Kate.

Samantha looks like she could be a model; she is tall and thin, with long dark-blonde hair. Kate grabs her arm and the three reunite.

Tyler walks up to Dad and says, "Hi, Grampa."

As he stands at the bed, I recall a similar moment years ago, but their places switched. *Luckily, we were in Arizona when Kate called to tell us Tyler was in the emergency room. Dad got us in the car and drove to California, straight to the hospital. I remember standing in the room, staring at Tyler in his white hospital gown with dark blue stripes, and Dad standing over him.*

I was always close with Kate's kids. Our connection is still strong, as the breaking of our forbearer drapes our souls with gloom.

Chloe, Curtis, and Cody walk in. We are united once again before the eyes of our creator, Dick. He says, "Curtis, you need to get one of those dollies so you can put me on it and wheel me around."

Curtis replies, "I don't know about that Pops."

Mom says, "Richard, you are not able to get out of the bed."

"What about at home, how will I get out of my chair?"

"There will be a bed where your chair is. You will be in the bed."

"How will I get to the bedroom?"

"You are not going to go to the bedroom. You will sleep in the bed, in the living room. You will be in the bed all the time."

"How will I get to the table for dinner?"

"You won't, you will eat in the bed. You can't get out of the bed, Richard. You don't have enough strength."

It is quiet for a while after that.

We finally decide to leave. I walk out of his room for the final time. I hit the number 447 on the door and say, "Goodbye, my sweet number, I'm sure we will meet again."

Back at the house, we converse about Dad.

I say, "What is so difficult is he still has so much hope, like the dolly and scooter ideas."

Tyler says, "I know, it's hard."

He would know, he watched his wife die a heartbreaking death. She was only 22.

We sit around the table and eat dinner. I ask Tyler, "Do you ever see your dad?"

He replies, "I see him all the time in me, and that's enough."

Isn't that the truth.

Before they leave, we move Dad's brown chair and some other things around to make room for the bed to arrive in the morning.

It's hard to imagine a hospital bed right in the middle of the goddamn living room.

Buddy runs out with something colored hot pink in his mouth.

"Oh my God, Buddy! That's my underwear!" Kate chases the dog, as the pink bottoms hang from his mouth.

We are laughing so hard we are crying. Kate finally gets them back. "Dammit Buddy, there's slobber all over them."

Day 10

It is mid-morning and I am in Mom's office on the computer, when I hear a man's voice, "Where is the bed going?"

There are still a few minutes left. Once the bed gets here, the core of this house will never be the same. Normally, I would be out there by now, curious, but I really want nothing to do with it. The clatter of the metal frame pierces through me. I'm intrigued of its construction, but I don't want to see what *he* looks like. *He, the one that builds the bed that holds this family captive.*

I become a hostage to mortality when I hear him say, "Okay, you are all set. Now let me show you how to use everything."

I hear the instructions, even though I am trying to block them out.

"Have a good day," he says, and the front door closes.

I walk out into the hallway and there is an oxygen machine. I follow its cord to the head of the bed that is sticking out in the hall. The long side of the bed is parallel to the fireplace with the foot of the bed about five feet in front of the television. I study the bed and can't believe what I see.

I say, "You've got to be kidding me, it's brown? Brown!"

Mom says, "I know. I thought that too."

Dad's favorite color is brown, and it drove Mom and me nuts.

I say, "This bed is ridiculous, it's ancient. How can it be brown? It has to be the first and last of this model ever made."

The bottom frame of the bed is brown. The mattress on top is a blue rectangular pad with folded white sterile sheets and the bed's remote piled on it. Silver metal, double bedrails line each side of the bed. Dad's end table, that used to be next to his chair, has a box of medical supplies on it. There is also a new table, a brown adjustable medical table with a slide out tray.

Mom walks over, "Come on Molls, help me put the sheets on the bed."

The phone rings. I answer it and hear, "Hi, this is Dr. Howard. I was calling because I want to recommend a few prescriptions for Richard."

"Oh, okay."

As I write, I wonder why he is giving him more medicine. I want to ask him if this isn't just prolonging everything, but I can't say it.

He says, "If he takes these and eats good meals he could make it 'till spring. It would be nice for him to see the warm weather."

He sure is hooked up on Dad seeing spring.

Spring always meant golf. Dad was cooped up all winter. He didn't do much but sit in his chair and watch television. However, there was always his putter and a club or two leaning against the wall. He would get up every so often and swing or putt balls into a cup. Golf Digest was always in his hand. He read the drills and then practiced the swings in the living room. As soon as spring came, he would take those swings to the course and try to repeat them. He spent spring, summer, and fall duplicating a smooth, deliberate, consistent attack of the golf ball. He was usually down the middle of the fairway. When he did get into trouble, he somehow got out easily and it never cost him too many shots.

The doorbell rings. Kate opens the door, and a woman greets us, "I'm Heather, your nurse from Angel Hospice."

She is not what I expected—much younger than I thought. We sit down at the table to begin our first lesson. I say to Heather, "The doctor called, and gave me more prescriptions. I thought his medicine was taken away."

She explains, "At the beginning, he needs to be on medications for anything causing complications. As time goes by, we will gradually take the medications away. You will want to read this book, it will tell you everything you need to know."

She opens the book. It is a big blue binder, and it is filled with death. Step by step, the process in complete detail and order—a death manual.

Basically, it's a yardage book. It's important to know all the possible shots, to be able to open a book and have it tell what trouble lies ahead. This book will guide Dad down these difficult fairways, and escort him home.

She flips the pages to the very back, and says, "This is his chart for his medications." She starts to fill it out while she continues, "These new ones, you will have to get today. Someone from hospice will be delivering the rest here tonight."

Mom asks, "So how many are there all together?"

Heather answers, "Looks like twenty-two. They all have different times and amounts. Some need to be taken with food and I marked food by those ones."

She hands Kate the chart.

Mom says, "Now, he can't have any morphine. He had it at the hospital, and he went totally berserk."

Heather replies, "Yes, I know. His chart specified that. In fact, it recommended he have no sedative drugs at all, which is very unusual in hospice. Eventually, he will have to have something to calm him down, but it definitely won't be morphine or anything close."

I ask, "Do you know of anybody for home care?"

Heather replies, "I know this great guy, Gabe."

The doorbell rings again.

I walk to the door and see the paramedic through the window. *Dad is home.* Kate and I quickly move the firewood from the walkway so the gurney can fit. I hear them turn the corner and move up onto the step. I'm hot, sweaty, and my eyes are blurry. I don't know why, but I'm upset.

Oh fuck it, just say something to him, Molly.

"Hi, Dad."

"Hi, Skeets."

They wheel him in the door. Mom says, "Hi, Richard."

He starts to cry, "I'm home, Tweets, I'm home."

The paramedics lift him off the gurney onto the bed.

He is so happy to be in the house, he actually looks like himself.

Mom signs off and Dad is officially delivered. Heather introduces herself to Dad. She asks him, "How do you feel?"

"I am so happy to be in my beautiful home."

"You do have a beautiful home," Heather replies.

She continues, "Okay, let's begin. He has to be rolled every couple hours."

She shows us how to use a folded sheet to roll him and move him when needed. She then says, "Let's see what's under here."

She takes off his tumor bandage. My eyes examine the big hole in the side of his chest, all the way under his arm. It looks like a poorly drawn circle. The tissue surrounding the tumor resembles a sponge that's falling apart. A substance of holes and crumbly pieces of inside stick out like a chunk of tuna casserole piled on a plate. The edges are hard and taught, but the center core is mushy and messy.

Heather shows me how to clean it with a spray bottle and gauze. She dabs it and then shapes a few pieces of gauze into a ball that she carefully fits inside the tumor's inner hole. She bandages it up and says, "You will want to do this twice a day, and check it for drainage. If it begins to drain a lot, you will want to change it more often."

As she lifts his arm trying to get the bandage taped, Dad yells out, "Damn, that hurts!"

"I'm sorry, I will be more careful with that."

She picks up the bedpan and asks, "Have you ever used one of these?"

Kate, Mom, and I shake our heads *no*.

The explanation didn't seem too difficult. Then again, it was just a trial run and not the real thing.

The bottoms of his feet have scabby open wounds from the nurses sliding him up and down the bed at the hospital. His left foot is turned in and his whole left leg is turning toward the other leg. This must be because he never had any therapy after the hip surgery. Heather tries to pull his feet apart, but the pain is too much. She says, "We can't let them link together, we need to separate them somehow."

She finds a small decorative pillow and says, "Okay Molly, I'm going to pull his feet apart, and you maneuver this in between them."

He screams out, but I get the task completed, and then put a second pillow between his legs to keep them from overlapping. Heather says, "With his tumor like that, the best thing for him to wear would be tee shirts cut up the back. This way you don't have to put anything over his head or really mess with the arm."

Mom says, "I will go get one."

Dad asks, "When can I sit in my chair?"

"You are staying in the bed," Kate responds.

Heather says, "You can do everything right from here. You will be very comfortable and don't have to move."

"What about when I shower?" Dad asks.

"Another nurse, Amy, will come to bathe you, so you don't have to get up to shower. You can remain relaxed right here and your family will make sure you are as comfortable as possible."

Mom walks up, "All right Richard, let me put this on you."

Heather picks up his arm and slides it through the sleeve easily, then picks up his other arm.

He shouts, "Ouch, that's my tumor one!"

Heather says, "Oh shoot, we need to be extra careful with that one."

She turns to Mom, "Well, I think that's everything. Please don't hesitate to call the hospice number and we can help you with any questions, no matter what time it is. I'll see you in the morning."

My eyes stick on her form. The door closes, and fear plagues my body.

Kate says to Mom, "You better go now and get those prescriptions, get it over with."

Mom walks over to the bed and says, "Now Richard, I am leaving. Do you have to go potty before I go?"

"No."

"Are you sure, because the girls are not going to be able to help you, and I won't be here."

"I don't have to go, Tweets. Now go to the store."

I hear the garage door close, and say to Kate, "Come on, let's go downstairs for a quick puff."

Kate hurries to follow me down the stairs. We inhale the herb, and breathe out our tensions. "Boy, did I need that. Much better," Kate says. "I should go check on him."

"Okay, I will be up in a minute."

My stomach is finally calm. I'm chilling, enjoying my moment when I hear Kate's voice, "Molly, Dad has to pee."

"What?"

"Dad has to pee."

"Are you kidding me?"

"No. Come on, he says he can't hold it."

I walk out of the bathroom and take a deep breath. It's *game time*. I run up the stairs at full force, reach the bed, and say, "Okay, I got this. I can do this. No problem."

"Good, because I can't," Kate says. "You better put gloves on."

"Right, gloves."

I get the pee bottle and try to pull his sweat pants down, but it's too hard. I say to Kate, "I need you to help me."

We are pulling our hardest, but we can't get his pants down past his butt. We laugh. No matter what we do, we can't move them. We finally get to his tighty-whities. I pull out his penis and put it in the bottle.

"Okay Dad, you can go now."

"You don't have it in right," he replies.

"Dad, it's in there."

"Molly, I'm telling you, it's not in there right. I'm gonna' pee all over the place."

"Dad, it is in there, I promise. Come on."

Kate encourages him, "It's okay, Dad, just go."

"Okay, I'm done," he tells us.

There is no pee in the bottle.

"I told you it wasn't in there," Dad complains.

I yell out, "Shit, there is pee all over the place. He is soaked. What the hell?"

"What? Are you serious?" Kate asks.

"God dammit! There is pee everywhere."

"We need to change him and get him out of these clothes," Kate says. "What a mess this is already."

"I have no idea what happened, it was in there."

Kate giggles, which makes me giggle, and now we can't stop laughing.

"Go find him some new underwear," Kate says.

I run to the bedroom. I open the dresser drawer I assume they are in.

"Socks!" I scream. "How in the fuck are there socks in this drawer?"

I open another drawer, "Oh my God! You've got to be kidding me."

I stick my hands into the multi-colored balls of rolled-up socks and clench their softness.

Kate yells, "What now?"

I open another drawer, grab the shirts and throw them over my head behind me. There are more round globes of fabric underneath the shirts. I am furious, tossing shirts out of the drawer until only different shades of pink and green socks are left in front of me.

Kate yells, "Molly, what are you doing?"

"This is ridiculous, I can't find any," I scream back.

I walk over to another dresser and open the bottom drawer.

"Finally! Why are they over here?"

I dart back out to the bed.

Kate and I are both sweating and panting as we finally get his pants down to his ankles. Dad says, "Oh, be careful, my feet."

We get the pants completely off. I throw them to the floor and say, "One done, one to go."

I put my hands on his underwear and begin to slide them down. However, they are too wet and not budging.

"How difficult can this be?" I scream out. "This is like the hardest thing I have ever done. I can't move them."

Kate tries to lift his ass up, but she can't even jiggle it. "Dad, can you lift your butt up a little so we can slide these off?"

"I'm trying, but this is the best I can do."

The underwear loosens and we finally get it off. I run to get a washcloth.

"The sheets are soaked," Kate says.

"Well, I have no idea how to change the sheet with him in the bed. We will have to wait until she gets back in the morning. I mean, we can't move him at all and we still have to put his new underwear on."

I dab his inner thigh and scrotum with the warm towel, "Okay, now let's get him dressed."

We get the underwear about halfway up his thigh, but we can't move them anymore. Once again, we are huffing and puffing. I wipe a bead of sweat off my cheek, and say, "That's it, I'm done. Mom can fix this when she gets home. Let's just cover him for now."

Kate says, "And leave him naked?"

"Well, no matter how hard we try, we can't get them on, so I give up."

"But he can't stay like this. His underwear are half on and he's, like, sticking out."

"Well, what do you suggest?"

"I guess I don't know either. Let's just cover him up and wait for Tweets."

We cover him with the blanket. I say, "I'm sorry Dad, but it's my first day on the job, and I'm just learning."

He snaps back, "I told you it wasn't in there."

I feel sad and embarrassed, as I make my way downstairs for a break from this nightmare.

I have no idea what I'm doing, and he should just be thankful that I'm trying.

Back upstairs, Kate is at the dining room table with a bottle of wine. I walk to the fridge and grab a beer.

We sit at the table in brief silence.

Dad hollers out, "You girls gonna' get drunk now?"

Kate replies, "Sure thinkin' about it."

I hear the garage door open, and say to Kate, "I hope she isn't going to be mad at us."

Mom walks in, notices our withered faces, and asks, "What happened now?"

I reply, "Well, we had some issues."

"What kind of issues?"

"Just go help him, please, you will see."

She walks over to him and says, "Richard, what did you do now?"

"I tried to tell them, Tweets."

I say to her, "You need to look under the blanket."

She lifts the blanket and bursts into laughter, "Geez and crackers, Molly, I'm gonna' pee my pants."

She crosses her legs, grabs her crotch, and runs into the bathroom. I say to Kate, "I'm glad she isn't mad."

She comes back out, and I tell her what happened. Kate says, "Let's see if the three of us can get his underwear pulled up."

I try to lift his butt as Mom and Kate try to slide on the underwear, but they just won't budge. He is too heavy.

Mom says, "I have to sit down."

I say, "Screw it, let's just leave it."

Kate and Mom both throw up their hands and say, "Fine."

We walk away, exhausted.

Mom gets dinner ready.

Kate and I stand next to the bed as Mom feeds him. She says, "How is it?"

He replies, "Delicious."

Kate says, "I bet it beats the hospital food."

I reply, "Yeah, but not the service. You just can't have both, huh, Dad?"

"I'm not complaining."

He ate all his food. He even asked for ice cream.

*

He is very needy. He complains about his feet throbbing all night. He asks us to rub them constantly.

Kate and Mom are in bed, and I stay on the couch next to him. I try to watch television, but he calls out my name, "Molly."

"Yeah, Dad."

"Will you rub my feet?"

This is going to be a long night.

I rub his feet and focus on keeping my eyes open. I am leaning back and forth, feeling like I've been standing here for hours, though only a few minutes have passed.

I ask him, "How's that Dad?"

"Good, that's good, Skeets, you can sit down."

I fall into the chair and turn my eyes to the television. Within a few minutes, I doze off.

"Molly, Molly," he yells out.

My eyes open slightly as I get up.

He asks, "Can you fix my pillow?"

I straighten it out. "Is that it Dad, do you need anything else?"

"I want some pop."

"Pop, okay, hold on."

I am walking to the kitchen ready to scream, and it hasn't even been twenty-five minutes since they went to bed.

I hand him his pop. "Okay Dad, let's go to sleep."

"Hold on Skeets, let me have a drink."

He presses the glass against his lips. He swallows and his lumpy Adam's apple struggles to force the liquid down his throat. It is a disturbing motion, setting me back to the age of four.

My years before eight took place in a different house. Our neighbor's across the street, Mabel and Carl, were an older couple, who babysat me all the time. One of my earliest memories is me in the driveway playing, and Mom running out of the house yelling, "Oh God, oh God, please. Molly, stay right here. Stay here, Molly!"

She ran across the street and into Mabel and Carl's house. My legs couldn't help but straighten. Deliberate little steps took me to their door, which was still wide open from when Mom ran in. I went through the den, then the kitchen. I got to the living room, and looked down the hall. I heard crying and sirens in the distance. I froze when I saw Mabel and Mom standing over Carl, who was lying on the bed. He was on his back and his hands and legs were very straight. The sirens were loud, and then they died off in front of the house. Mabel's arms flared down to the bed, as she collapsed and screamed, "Carl, no, no, please. God, no."

Carl's body was still and non-responsive. The bed was shaking from her cries, but Carl was limp, lifeless, motionless, dead. Guys in tight blue tee shirts and baggy yellow overalls ran by me. I couldn't see what was going on. They were blocking my view of the bed. I walked toward them, but I heard Dad's voice, "Come on Skeets, you shouldn't be here."

His hands were strong on my sides as he swooped me up. I tucked myself in his chest, and his arms wrapped around me. He shuffled me through the house, and back across the street. My eyes were full of tears. Dad's body felt warm; he was sweaty and nervous. We got in the house and ended up in front of the fridge. He opened the door and grabbed a can of soda. He took a big, long gulp. My eyes were centered on his Adam's apple as it effortlessly slid up and down his throat. He took a deep breath, "Here ya' go Skeets, have a sip of pop."

He put the can to my lips and I wrapped my fingers around it. I took a sip and let the cool, sweet, flavor swish around in my mouth. He closed the fridge and said, "Let's see what's on TV, Skeets."

Standing at his side almost thirty years later he says, "Molly, Molls, I'm done with my pop."

I grab the glass from his wrinkly, fragile grip, "Okay Dad, let's go to sleep now."

"Skeets, but can we watch TV for a bit?"

"Sure Dad, but please just try to be still."

I lie down on the couch. The noise of the television puts me right back to that day, the day Carl died.

With the can of soda tight in my hands, Dad carried me out of the kitchen to the living room. He sat me down on the couch and then proceeded to his chair. He never said anything. We sat there for a long time. His terrified silence then, I had forgotten, until now.

Buddy climbs up next to me and we fall asleep for a good thirty minutes.

Dad's voice wakes me, "Molly, I have to pee."

I walk down the hallway like a zombie, and yell out, "Mom!"

She yells back, "What?"

"Dad has to pee."

She comes out, and he pees his first of five pees for the night. I get both of them up twice to turn him. He has had about seven sips of pop, four foot massages, and five or six pillow fluffs. When I finally feel like he is about to sleep he says, "Molly, I want an orange."

It's 3:38 a.m., as I walk to the kitchen. Of course, the oranges are in the garage and it is fucking freezing out there.

I stand at the counter, peeling the orange, thinking how ridiculous this is. I look at Buddy, who is sitting, watching me, "Can you believe this? I am cutting up tiny baby orange bites at three in the morning."

I feed Dad the orange bites, one at a time. He chews, and chews, and finally we get to the last one. I say, "Now Dad, this is it. You need to go to sleep."

Day 11

It is still dark when I open my eyes to his words, "Molly, get your mom up."

"Dad, it's only 6:20. It's too early. Mom needs her sleep. Now, let's sleep for a couple more hours."

About ten minutes later, he asks again, "Molly, wake up your mom."

I ignore his plea, and he is silent, but only for about another ten minutes.

He yells, "Molly, I'm not going to ask you again, now please go get Mom."

Kate walks out and says, "Dad you need to let her sleep."

He responds, "I'm hungry."

"Okay, what do you want?" I ask him.

"Honey Nut and a cookie."

I am looking for the cereal in the pantry, but having a hell of a time finding it. The pantry is full of empty stuff; boxes and jars with barely anything left in them.

I ask Kate, "Have you seen this?"

She says, "I know, come over here."

I walk over and follow her to the fridge. She opens it. "Look at this."

There are at least ten salad dressing bottles, all turned upside down. She picks one up and says, "They are all just like this."

The bottle has, maybe, two drops left in it.

Mom walks from the hall, into the living room, and straight towards us in the kitchen as she says, "Dad likes his cereal a certain way."

I reply, "Then you can do it because I can't find anything."

I dart to the stairs and slip away. In the bathroom, in the corner of the basement, I regain my sanity. Marijuana smoke rings entertain me; they are a distraction from my agitated thoughts. I'm angry, but I don't know why. Soon I'm pretty high, and curious about what's going on up there. I take one more puff, look into the mirror, and blow out. Smoke fills the glass and my face evaporates. I laugh, run to the stairs, and sprint up them.

Mom is having a difficult time feeding Dad. He is spilling, and she is not happy.

"Richard, open your mouth. Come on, what are you doing?" she says.

He is still chewing, as he screams out, "I'm eating, Tweets. I'm eating."

"God, Dick, you are so slow."

"I'm an old fart. I'm not young like you, Tweets."

"Well, you had a good life, a very good life."

He takes forever to eat his cereal. After that, he wants a bagel, and then an orange. He tops it all off with a couple of cookies.

The doorbell rings. It's Heather. She takes all his vitals and then starts on the tumor. I watch her the best I can. Mom is outside, and all of a sudden Buddy runs in with the neighbor's dog, Wrigley. He is an adorable black and white Shih Tzu with a snaggle-tooth. The dogs are going crazy, chasing each other.

Mom is yelling, "Wrigley's here! Wrigley's here!"

She doesn't even acknowledge what's going on at the bed.

I get the dogs back outside and close the door.

Heather says, "We need to change the sheets."

We are all standing at the bed as she pulls the blanket off and his *everything* is sticking out. Kate quickly pulls down his shirt, "I forgot we left him like that."

"We had some issues last night," I say.

We laugh as Mom tells the story.

Changing the sheets takes all four of us to do it this first time. Kate and I hold him on his side while Heather and Mom roll the sheet under him as much as they can. Then we roll him to his other side to get the sheet out from underneath him. Sweat is pouring out of me as I say, "He is heavy."

Heather responds, "He will get heavier, too. Now, do you want to put pants on him?"

I reply, "No, he is done with pants and underwear."

Mom and Kate agree that the blanket is good enough.

Heather says, "You do what's easiest for you, you are the ones doing it."

She gets ready to leave.

"Now, tomorrow you are on your own, Thursday morning Amy will be here, and I will be back on Friday."

I must have a look of panic because she says, "You will be fine. You can call anytime."

"Easy for you to say, you do it every day," I moan.

"You will be all right, don't worry. See you Friday."

I'm exhausted; it's finally quiet in the house. I lie down on the couch to rest my eyes, but I hear the door open.

Lily says, "Hello, I'm here to get my Buddy."

She gets one arm out of her jacket, her head pops up, and she sees *The Scene*. She freezes in the foyer, a hardwood path from the door that leads to the carpet, indicating the edge of the living room. She looks over Mom's pink recliner, past the pink-flowered couches, and her eyes settle on the bed.

"He's home. Dick, you're home."

She finishes with her jacket, but her view is fixed.

The gray of his hair glistens through the steel rails that hold him secure.

She approaches The Scene as her hands reach out to the bars and grab them firmly, "Hi Dick, how are you feeling?"

"Lily, is that you?"

"I bet you are glad to be home."

"I have never been happier, Lily."

I ask Lily, "How was Jamaica?"

"It was great, we met some good people from Michigan. But then your uncle and them scored some pot.

Mickey thought he could handle it but it knocked him on his ass. We got in the biggest fight because he could barely move for a day."

Kate and I laugh. "See Mom, Mickey smoked weed in Jamaica."

Mom yells, "I don't want to hear about it, that's my brother."

"Well then, be glad you weren't there, Tweedy," Lily says. "All right Dick, I need to take Buddy home, but we will be back this weekend."

I hug Buddy tightly, kiss him, and say, "Bye Bud. You be a good boy."

Buddy, helped me out at night. The last couple nights he has slept on the couch with me. He makes me feel safe.

The door opens again. It's Babe and Henry, Wrigley's parents, from across the street. They have been in the neighborhood almost as long as we have. When I lived here they never did anything with Mom and Dad, but in the last few years they have become close. Babe was thin, but now, stocky. Henry has a scruffy beard, and honestly, except for the glasses, looks nothing like I recall. He isn't even in the door, before his eyes attach to The Scene.

Babe says, "We brought you an air mattress, so you can sleep next to him."

I reply, "Oh, that's great, it will be much easier."

Henry is still not in the door. Babe turns her head, and grabs the back of the couch. She recovers, and her hands slide into the pockets of her form-fitting black leather coat as she confidently walks toward the bed, and says, "Hi Dick."

Dad's eyes go up, "Hi Babe."

Henry somehow gets to the bedrails before Babe, and says, "Hi Weasel, you glad to be home?"

Dad smiles, "Henry, I can't tell you how happy I am to be home. It's absolutely wonderful."

Henry shrugs his shoulders and grins, "That's great Dick. You got a great set up here."

Kate and I inflate the mattress, and I try it out. Everyone is talking, but I am dozing off when the door opens again. Leslie walks in and says, "Hello."

She pauses, tilts her head to the side, and smiles as she approaches Dad.

She ends up staying until everyone else leaves.

We are turning Dad for the third time, trying to position pillows to his liking. He says, "Please fix my crack, it's killing me."

"He probably has a bed sore down there somewhere," Leslie says.

Perfect. It just gets more interesting as the minutes go by.

Kate and I turn him on his side toward us, while Leslie doctors him up.

Leslie says, "Yeah, he has a very small sore but it is in a very sensitive area. Imagine having a paper cut right in your butt crack."

We finally sit down, but within a minute Dad says, "I have to pee."

Leslie says, "I got it, that's why I'm here."

As she assists him she says, "I bet you never thought I'd be doing this, huh, Dick?"

He doesn't respond.

What is he thinking? What is going through his mind as he lies there? He sure doesn't say much, for someone who is about to die.

Curtis walks in the front door at 5:15 p.m. His eyes hit The Scene, and his movement stops. Chloe, eager to see her grandpa, without pause, walks to his side and says, "Hi Gramps, how does it feel to finally be home?"

His eyes are big and blue, "It's wonderful, just wonderful."

Curtis advances, "Hey Pops, you're home, and done with that hospital place."

Dad turns his head and looks up as Curtis approaches the bed. Curtis's hands are in his coat pockets, but when he reaches the rails, his right hand extents out to Dad's shoulder and his left hand clutches the silver steel.

Dad says, "I hated that horse-bittle."

"I know Dad, I know you're happy to be home."

Curtis laughs and hollers, "Pops is *happy*, happy to be home."

*

Mom and Kate are in bed. Dad keeps calling me over, complaining about pain.

He says, "It's so hot in here, Molly."

"Okay, Dad. What do you want me to do?"

Kate and Mom come out to see what all the fuss is about.

I say, "Dad is getting me up every few minutes."

Mom says, "He doesn't look good to me."

I reply, "Something ain't right."

Kate and Mom decide to sleep out here with me.

He yells out, "Katie, will you rub my feet?"

She sluggishly gets up and walks over.

I close my eyes and try to calm down. Suddenly, I realize, I'm going to get sick, and run to the bathroom. I stare at the water against the white of the bowl.

What is going on here? What is the purpose of this moment, this day, this situation? It doesn't matter. I'm here, and it is happening. Get up, get out there, and deal with it.

I rise from the floor and make my way to the downstairs bathroom. I sit down on the cold tile floor, as I inhale the reefer. Thank God I have some. It takes me a lot of deep breaths, and a few puffs, but I finally feel better. I make my way up the stairs, saying, "God, please, just take him tonight. Please, Lord."

I lie back down on the couch.

Mom asks, "Are you okay?"

"Yeah."

"Now Kate is in there with the runs," she says.

"Ma! Ma, hey Ma!" Dad screams out.

"What, Richard?"

"Take me to bed."

"You are in bed."

"Oh come on, Ma, would you please take me to bed?"

"Richard, that is your bed, you are not going anywhere. You are sleeping there. Now go to sleep."

He screams out, "God dammit Tweets, don't be such a donkey nuts. Why can't you just put me to bed?"

We explain to him why he can't get out of the bed. Mom says, "Richard, you will never be able to get out of that bed."

This goes on for hours.

He finally moves on to another topic, "Please rub my feet, Tweets, they are on fire."

Day 12

The sun shines through the window and into my eyeballs.

How many more nights can this go on?

"Molly, Molly!" he yells.

I ignore him. I don't want to move for anything.

"Ma, Ma," he screams.

I hear Mom's weary voice, "What is it, Dick?"

"I'm hungry."

"Fine Dick, I will get your breakfast ready."

Mom is feeding him, and he asks, "When do I get to take my shower?"

She replies, "You aren't going to take a shower. Someone will be here tomorrow to bathe you."

"How am I going to get out of the bed to take a shower?"

"You are not going to get out of the bed, Dick."

"What about my radiation?"

"You are done with it."

"So, I am just going to lay here and die?"

Nobody says a word. Kate and I look at each other.

Mom says, "There's nothing they can do for your tumor. You know that, Richard."

There is silence for a while. I am trying to focus on the television, anything other than what is going on.

Kate says, "We need to do the tumor."

I put on the teal green gloves, and gently peel the tape from his wrinkly pale skin. I pull off the gauze, making my way to the inner hole. My fingers grab a ball of gauze that had been stuffed into the tumor. It unravels and brown spongy particles cling to the soft white cloth. Holding the flesh-specked gauze, I say, "I can't stand the smell, it's making me gag. I need to get spray."

Kate says, "Okay, go ahead, let's let it breathe a little."

I run into the bathroom and open the cabinet. There are tons of sprays. I grab one; it's empty. I grab another, but it is empty too. I grab another, and another, and another—they are all empty.

I scream out, "Oh my God, you are killing me! Why do you keep these?"

"There is a new one in the laundry room, on the sink," Mom screams back.

I run through the house singing, "Crazy, crazy, my Midwestern mother is crazy."

I spray the entire bottle throughout the house before approaching The Scene to finish my task. Kate hands me the spray bottle of cancer cleaner, and with the tip of my finger pressing the trigger, little white bubbles appear, and take over the dryness of the diseased chamber. I look inside, deeper, and see the inner tunnel of the carcinoma, filled with fluid; canals of green poison, flow alongside red suds of blood that still remain for the fight.

The front door opens, I hear Aunt Susan, "Hello, we got your stuff, and Dick, I got you your chocolate bar."

The gallery is filling.

Aunt Susan is my mom's sister. She is bubbly, and

always smiling in a silly kind of way. She makes her way to the kitchen with a bag of groceries. Her response to The Scene is quite casual compared to the ones before her.

Her husband, Uncle Jake, is now through the door. He stands still with his hands in his coat pockets and surveys the room.

Aunt Susan approaches Dad and says, "Here Dick, you want some chocolate?"

"Yeah, sounds good," he says.

She breaks off a piece, and hands it to him, "Here you go."

Dad says, "Is Jake here?"

Uncle Jake is still at the door.

"Yeah, I'm here Dick."

He finally makes his way to The Scene, but nowhere near the rails, "So, you glad to be out of that horrible hospital and back home?"

"I've never been happier, Jake. I hated that horse-biddle."

"Yeah, those hospitals are awful, I won't go near them," Jake says, with his hands still in his pockets.

A few hours have gone by before our next pair of fans walks through the door. It is a slow process, for Aunt Judy's legs are wobbly and her cane not confident. Shelly, behind her, helps take off her jacket.

Shelly is one of Mom's best friends. Since I can remember, she and her husband, Eddie, have been around. Shelly is always cheery, her dimples glow off her chubby cheeks. But she has never encountered a scene like this coming through the door.

She whimpers, "My little Weasel, you are home, my little Weasel."

She hurries to his side, grabs his hand, and says, "Weasel, are you happy to be home, my sweetheart?"

"Shell's, I can't tell you how happy I am to be home. Where's the Big Ed?"

"He isn't here. I brought your sister instead, and left him at home."

"Good thinking. Sis, you here?"

Aunt Judy yells, "Yeah, I'm getting there."

She grabs the bed rail. Kate puts a chair behind and helps her sit down.

"How are you doing, Bro? You feel better, now you're home?"

"Much better, so much better, Sis, it's great. I just can't tell ya' how wonderful it is."

Aunt Judy sits with him, as we play a game of Hand and Foot.

I watch them at the bed.

I never had a sibling; I grew up mostly alone. I never realized their bond until now. They have been together since they can remember – childhood, business, and now a deathbed. Is this the last conversation they will have? Another piece will be taken from her life; another bed she sits beside, and waits for the falling of a man.

After a while, Shelly says, "We have to get going."

Aunt Judy eventually gets up and says, "Okay Bro, I love you very much."

She leans in and kisses him. He replies with a stutter, "I love you too, Sis."

Shelly says, "My little Weasel, I'm gonna' miss you, Weasel."

He replies, "I'm gonna' miss you too, Shells."

That's the first time anyone has made reference to his departure, and he even acknowledged it.

As they walk out the door Shelly yells, "Bye, Weasel."

Dad yells back, "Bye, Shells."

*

It's late and we are finally alone, sitting around the table, eating dinner, but Dad's voice makes it difficult.

"Molly, will you move my pillow up?"

Mom replies, "Dick, we are trying to eat, now let your daughter be."

I get a few bites in.

"Molly, Kate, will someone please help me."

I yell back, "Dad, I know for a fact you waited way longer in the hospital when you needed something."

"Yeah, but you are my family, you are supposed to take care of me."

Kate chuckles, "Oh man, poor Dad."

"Oh Richard, you always got what you wanted. God, you are a piece of work," Mom hollers.

*

I walk into the kitchen to get Dad some pop, and the digits 11:47 glare at me.

It is going to be another fabulous night.

This is only his first request, but then again, Mom and Kate only went to bed eight minutes ago.

"Okay Dad, here is your pop, take a sip."

As he sips it, he spills it all over himself. Before I realize what I am saying, I yell out, "God dammit, Dad."

He barks back, "You are the one who took it away from me when I was still drinking, let me finish."

Every little task is becoming difficult. His turtle-like habits remind me of his golf game. Time was not of importance when he was hitting the golf ball. He had this never-ending set-up before he swung the club. He would dance with his feet as he looked back and forth from the ball down to his target, shifting up and down, while firming his stance. This pre-shot routine was over forty-seconds long, slower than most golfers, but he didn't care. He knew he was slow, and no matter the circumstance, he never hurried. His death is similar, with a delay, a hesitation before he trusts his swing.

I lie back down and stare at the television.

"Molly," he whispers.

"Yeah, Dad."

"Will you rub my feet?"

I want to say *no* more than anything, but I can't. I get up and meet his command.

He finally says, "Okay, let's go to sleep now."

"Oh Dad, that would be great."

I turn off the television.

Could this be, he actually wants to sleep?

My eyes shut for a good seven minutes, and then his voice pierces, "I have to pee."

My mouth reacts to his plea, "Are you kidding me? You have to pee? You have to pee? Are you sure, Dad, you have to pee?"

He screams out, "Yes, I have to pee. Now come on, hurry up, Molly."

I am just kneeling, not yet all the way standing when I hear footsteps coming down the hall.

"I'm coming Dick, I'm coming," Mom hollers out.

She walks in and she is not looking too happy. She says to him, "Now Richard, you need to go to sleep. Molly needs to get some sleep. You think you could let your daughter sleep?"

"Tweets, I have to pee."

"This is it. No more. Do you hear me, Dick? Dick, do you hear me?"

He does not reply. She finally finishes with him, and says again, "Richard, do you understand me?"

"Yes, Tweedles. Now go to bed, Tweets," he answers.

Mom yells back, "You're the one who needs to go to bed."

She turns off the light, "Now go to sleep. Don't be so naughty."

I cover myself completely in the blanket and bury my head under the pillow. I thought I could block out his voice of want for the rest of the night.

"Molly, Molly, what time is it?"

"It is only 12:40 Dad, let's try to get some sleep."

"Okay, Molls."

He lies awake all night, scared to close his eyes. He waits for sunlight, and when the silence is too much he calls out my name. His requests are not important but they force me to stand by him. He does this purely for comfort. The warmth of my existence enables him to know he is still in existence too. Even though I lie right beside him, he is completely alone.

His voice is strong when he asks, "What time is it?"

I do not respond.

A few moments later, he is a bit louder, but whimpers out, "Molly."

I still do not respond. I want to test him, to see how far he will go, even though I know he will call me until I oblige.

I understand he is failing, but there is more to dying than requesting and getting whatever you want. He did that all his life. We allowed him to, and now we let him take advantage of us again. I'm obviously his nurse, that's how he treats me, and so that's how I will act in return.

Now he lets out an irritated howl, "Molly, Molly, Molly, Molly, Molls."

I scream out, "What Dad, what now?"

"What time is it?"

I rip the covers off of my head and look up at the clock. I yell back, "It's almost 3:30. It's still early. We need to sleep. We have a big day tomorrow."

There is no response from his weary lips.

I pull the covers back over my head, but my name once again crawls off his tongue, "Molly."

I respond immediately this time, "Yeah Dad, what is it?"

"Why is tomorrow a big day?"

"The Pastor is coming tomorrow. That's why it is important we get our rest."

"Okay, well let's go to sleep, Skeeters."

"Yeah, let's go to sleep. We need to be ready when the Pastor gets here."

I actually may have shut him up for the rest of the night. I know he will now think about the Pastor's visit. He wonders if the Pastor can free his soul of sorrow.

I believe we've just set a record. It's over an hour before his mouth is active again, "Molly, where is Mom?"

I deny his inquiry, but he yells out again, "Molly, get your mom."

I whisper back, "Dad, she is asleep. Let her sleep."

"But the Pastor is coming, we need to get up. She needs to get ready."

"Oh Dad, come on. It is only 4:15, and we need to sleep for another few hours. We really need to get some sleep. Please, Dad."

Another calculating play, he uses my own words against me, turning the Pastor's visit into getting what he wants – the night vanished. He is a slippery little weasel. Maybe if he pitied the ones he hurt, his transgressions would be forgiven. Then again, he is the kind of man who only pities himself.

"Okay Molly, you can get Mom up now."

My eyes open and a foggy light shines through the blanket. "Dad, it is only six, so we have a couple more hours."

"The Pastor likes to come early. You need to get Mom

up, now."

"No. Now go to sleep. Mom needs her rest. I can't have her at risk too. Now let her sleep."

Fifteen minutes later he says, "I have to pee."

"Fine, I'm done anyway."

I get up, walk down the hall, and yell, "Mom!"

She says, "I'm coming."

I lie back down on the mattress.

He asks, "Will you fix my crack, Tweets?"

"Oh Dick, what's wrong with your crack?"

"It hurts. It hurts like a mother-fucker, and I'm asking you to fix it for me."

"Boy, are you naughty."

"I'm in pain, Tweets, I'm in pain, and I'm asking you as my wife to help me."

"There is only so much we can do. Dick, you have to understand."

I add, "You are home. You could be in the nursing home. Would you rather be there?"

"No."

"Well, then you need to just deal with what you got here. Us. Now, we will roll you and try to get you comfortable, but then you have to go to sleep."

Kate walks out. "Okay, let's try to fix this crack issue."

We roll him and Mom asks, "Now, how is that, Pa?"

He sighs, "Oh, much better."

Mom says, "I'm going to lie back down for a little bit. Now, let's try to sleep for another couple hours."

Kate and Mom walk back to their bedrooms.

I tell Dad I have to go to the bathroom and fly downstairs.

I am stoned solid as I walk back upstairs. His eyes are closed. He seems to be asleep. In slow motion, I maneuver myself onto the mattress and allow my body to sink in.

I'm asleep, until I hear Kate in the kitchen making coffee. Dad's eyes are still closed. I put the blanket over my head, but his voice does not allow much more rest, as he says, "Is someone going to get Mom up?"

"Why do you want her up so bad?" I ask.

"It's mornin', don't people get up in the mornin'?"

I don't respond. I know I cannot win.

He moves onto another demand, "I want an orange. Skeeters, will you get me an orange?"

Mom walks out and says, "Dick, are you ready for breakfast?"

He replies, "Yeah, I want Honey Nut, an orange, and two cookies,"

As she walks into the kitchen and begins his order, she hollers at him, "Dick, do you want a bagel?"

He yells back, "Yes."

I need another break. What little patience I was given, is about to be gone.

I say to Mom, "I need to go brush my teeth."

*

The doorbell rings; it's the aide, who looks to be in her early 20s. "Hi, I'm Amy."

She walks confidently to the bed, and sets her bag on the floor.

"Hello, I'm Amy. How are you feeling this morning?

Dad says, "I need to take a shower."

She replies, "Well, I'm going to give you a bath, how about that?

"You are?"

"Yep, I just have to get some water."

She looks at Mom and asks, "Where can I fill this?"

She pulls a little blue plastic tub out of her bag.

"You can use the utility sink in the laundry room," Mom says, pointing.

Amy walks back to the bed with the tub filled with water and soap. She takes off his shirt. She notices the bandage and asks, "Does this need to be cleaned?"

I reply, "Oh yeah, do you do that?"

She says, "I can, but did they show you how?"

I reply, "Yes."

She responds, "If you show me how, I will help you."

I walk over to the bed and we begin. She takes the bandage off, and I find myself examining the wound. Kate is right here helping. As disgusting as it is, it is intriguing as well.

I say to Amy, "I hope the smell doesn't get any worse. I don't do well with smells. I have walked by a coffee shop and the smell made me sick to my stomach."

Amy responds, "It will get worse. You should put Vicks under your nose."

She is right, the smell will get worse, the tumor will get worse, and this whole situation is going to get worse.

Kate lifts his arm, as I try to wrap it up.

He yells, "God dammit, that hurts."

"I'm sorry Dad, I am trying to be as gentle as I can."

"Okay Skeets, that's enough. No more, now leave me alone."

I say to Amy, "It's very difficult because he won't let me move his arm away from his side."

She replies, "Do what you can, and when he starts to get frustrated, just stop for a moment. Give him a couple minutes before you continue."

Amy is quite helpful, and finds her way around like she lives here; I wish she did.

*

I finally get in the shower. The water is hard and thick as it hits my skin. It feels great to be the farthest away possible from the site of distress my eyes see constantly.

I walk up the stairs and hear a man's voice. As I get closer, I realize it is Pastor. I walk in and he says, "Hello Molly,"

"Hi Pastor."

"So you must like it out there in California?" he teases.

Mom interjects, "Oh she loves it. She would never come back here. She thinks we are all crazy."

Pastor replies, "My daughter says she will never come back here either."

I say, "When you move away from here you realize a world exists that is open to all beliefs, and not just the one of the land."

Pastor smirks, "So you Californians do whatever you want?"

"Exactly, but what is important; we do it without being judged."

"Reminds me of when my daughter came home with her tattoo."

"See, a perfect example. People here think people with tattoos are bad—Devil worshiping people."

Mom yells, "Molly, that's not true."

I reply, "What about Chloe? You always used to comment about her tattoos. Now you don't say anything. You know why? Because you learned who she is beneath the skin, and you don't judge her due to her appearance anymore."

Mom in a high pitch, sulking tone says, "Oh, Molly."

"Well, am I right?"

She sighs, "Oh Molls, you sure aren't like your Mother, that's for sure."

Pastor walks to The Scene, "Hi Dick."

"Hi Pastor."

"How are you feeling?"

"I'm tired, but I can't sleep at night."

"Do you pray?"

"Yeah, but you should pray, you're the Pastor."

"Okay, well, let's pray."

Mom, Kate, and I proceed to the bed. Our hands clench together to form the perfect circle. Pastor begins, "Dear Lord, we thank you for bringing Richard home, and ask you to bless him and his family. Lord, please watch over and protect this house. Give them the strength to prepare Richard for your kingdom. Lord, please give us the courage to destroy fear and announce our faith in you. In your almighty name, Amen."

Amen echoes around The Scene, as Pastor lets go of my hand.

Pastor asks, "So Kate, how long are you staying?"

She replies, "I'm not sure yet, probably first of next week."

This is going to be difficult without Kate – Mom, Dad, and me, in the house, alone, in an unbearable situation. Knowing a life is about to end fills this house with hesitation, because nobody knows how to embrace a fearful soul.

Pastor is getting ready to leave, "Kate, have a safe trip back to California, where everyone does whatever they want."

Mom laughs, "Yeah, right."

I say, "You know what the difference is between the Midwest and California? In the Midwest everyone cares about what everyone else thinks. In California, nobody gives a shit."

Mom yells out, "Molly!"

"Well, it's true. If we could meet in the middle somewhere, we would have a decent society."

Shaking her head up and down, Kate chuckles, "I agree."

Pastor isn't even out the door a few seconds, and Dad hollers out, "Is it time for lunch?"

Mom yells back from the kitchen, "What do you want, Dick?"

"What are my choices?"

"What about a ham sandwich?"

"Okay. Toasted."

I sit in the chair with my eyes barely open. Kate sinks in her chair so deeply only a crowbar could get her out.

Mom is feeding him the sandwich as she cries out, "Geez and crackers, what a mess, Richard you are getting crumbs everywhere."

Dad yells out, "I need a sip of pop."

His table is filled with empty glasses.

I walk into the kitchen, and Mom calls after me, "You have to get a new bottle from outside."

I walk into the garage and open the side door. Standing in the threshold, bright white is all I see. My eyes are squinting, and the chill of the air is harsh on my skin. New air hasn't hit my nose in a few days.

This is the freshest air I have ever felt.

The snow is too white for my weak eyes, my head begins to ache, and I close the door.

When will I again be more than just a few feet away from freedom? Our lives have been taken over by a fading man who has no compassion for anyone except himself.

Back in the house, I pour the soda into the glass, and a tear runs down my cheek. The brightness of the snow's reflection was hard on my eyes. The strain on my lids has become too much, they need to close.

I walk over to The Scene. Mom is still trying to shove the sandwich into his mouth, and he takes the biggest bite he can.

I laugh, "You can't just give him the whole sandwich. It's too much for him. He could choke. You didn't even cut it in half."

Mom ignores me as she says to him, "Geez and crackers, Richard, you are making a mess."

With a mouthful he mumbles, "I need a sip."

I reply, "Okay, well chew it all and swallow it first."

His chewing makes me want to stick a twig in my eye; it is the most measured procedure of such a simple task I've ever seen.

Mom blurts out, "What are you doing, Dick?"

He still is chewing. At last he swallows and says, "Oh Tweets, don't be such a donkey nuts. I'm eating. I'm slow, I'm not fast like you."

She stuffs the rest of the sandwich in his mouth. I sit down, for I know it will take him at least a few minutes to get that hunk down.

It's exactly three minutes later when he says, "Molly, I need a sip."

As I get up, he says, "A couple cookies too, Molls."

The door opens and Leslie walks in.

"Thank God," I say.

She says to me, "Molly, you look so tired, you need to get some sleep."

"I'm going downstairs right now to take a nap," I say, and run down the stairs. About a third of the way down, I jump through the air over the remaining steps and land solidly on my feet. The ceiling is low and the stairs are steep, but I have never missed that jump.

I lie down without interruption, it's nice and dark. The couch embraces me, as I curl up into a ball and close my eyes. At the same time, I am uncomfortable being distant from The Scene.

What happens next will be the last of his recollections. From this time on I will live without a Dad.

I hear pounding footsteps coming from upstairs and my eyes open. I see the clock, and it has been almost three hours.

I better get up there and see what is going on. First, I will go to the bathroom and prepare.

The downstairs bathroom has become my sanctuary and my sanity. This is my break from the burden that swarms this entire house—the wait for death. I have no choice but to leave the little serenity that this space gives me. I take my last puff as though it is the last sip of water on a long desert journey.

Back upstairs, I look at him, and I know he believes he is going straight to hell. As the hours go by, the three of us cater to his every need, including rubbing his feet, feeding him ice cream, hydrating him, basically, doing everything possible to make him comfortable. All he does is complain, unless, of course, he needs a cookie.

Before I know it, Kate and Mom are in their rooms, and I am alone with my dying father. I decide to submerse myself into the figures on the television, and pretend I am there and not here.

However, before I can even try to understand what's on the screen, he whimpers, "Molly."

I sigh, "Yeah Dad."

"Can you fix my pillow?"

Here begins another night of meaningless requests, made to silence the whispers of death. I don't know what to do; an easy-going chat cannot exist between us. Talking to him about something - anything - would help, but I can't think of anything that isn't complicated.

He is restless between his sheets and the sound irritates me. "Hey Dad, are you awake?"

"Yeah Skeeters, I can't sleep."

"You need to try, Dad, close your eyes and drift off."

His voice crackles, "But Molls, my eyes won't close."

"It's okay Dad, just close them, everything is going to be okay, I promise, just go to sleep."

"I will try, Skeeters."

No shot is easy, but his are extremely difficult. The terrain is uneven and full of hazards. The grass is thick where he lies. Errant shots have put him in dangerous positions. The shot at hand is always the most important, understanding where the ball will land, and how it effects the execution of the shot after that, is critical. Making sure the first shot doesn't end up in front of trouble for the second shot, and so on, and so on. Seeing what's ahead is not always an option, but this doesn't mean it is not worth looking. Wrong shots will be repeated. Knowing in the moment that they will affect the rest of the game, doesn't always mean that changes are attempted. Sometimes realization doesn't set in until the end, when the score is totaled.

All through the night, I can hear Mom coughing to the point of vomit.

Plus, I have been awakened at least ten times with the question, "Molly, what time is it?"

Finally, light begins to shine through the house. It is dawn, and he outlasted the darkness once more.

"Dad, it is still early. It isn't even six."

"It's morning, get your mom up."

"Dad, Mom was up all night coughing. This situation is already too much stress on her. Now go to sleep for another couple hours."

I close my eyes and somehow fall asleep.

It's about 9:30 a.m. when the temples in my skull begin to vibrate again.

I pull the blanket off my face when I hear Mom's voice, "You will never get out of this bed."

"But Tweets, I need to take a shower."

"Richard, you are not taking a shower. Now, what do you want for breakfast."

"Eggs and Honey Nut with toast."

"Okay, now be quiet, your daughters are still sleeping. Please Richard, be good while I get your food."

"Okay Tweets, but can I have a cookie to hold me over?"

This situation is above my head. I need some help here. I should contact the one person who always saves me, my best friend Rebecca.

I send her a text that says:

Whatever little faith I had in God, I'm losing. Why is God making him suffer? Making us all suffer? He has so much hope. Why do I have to tell him he has to die?

Rebecca responds:

We live in a fallen world because of man's free will. God never said this life would be easy. He only promises your eternity to be secure. If you trust him, eternity is forever. I'd start trusting him over anything else. Stop messing around, Molly, life is hard and short.

Oh boy, after reading that response, I know, she will be sending many more.

Another one arrives:

First of all, God is good. Our pain is because Adam and Eve chose to eat from the tree of good and evil. This was not God's plan for anyone to suffer. We have a redeemer. It's Jesus, and he is the only way to be saved. Your dad will die. Everyone dies. Lots of people suffer. It sucks, but his best bet right now is to put faith in the Lord, so he will be in Heaven and have eternal peace. Talk to him, Molly, if you love him, because Hell is real suffering.

Blah, blah, blah, I can't take her nonsense. What was I thinking?

Her words keep coming:

No one has to tell him he is going to die. The will in all of us is very strong. Knowing he is dying is not the concern, but where he is going is what you should be worried about. You can still talk to him about it, even if he has ten more years.

I am getting mad. This is not something I understand, nor do I want to. Rebecca always was an outspoken Christian. We have had many arguments throughout the years over our different beliefs, but miles away from the situation, she understands it completely. I can't come to terms with what she is telling me. I wasn't looking for a preacher, and I will ignore her advice.

I debate the theory of God and the Bible. To me, it is just a book written by a bunch of drunks wanting to screw with generations to come. Some people buy into it, some people don't. I'm sure not one to follow any book. I think people who believe a book, and actually live according to it are fools. It is just a book, and the author is not named God.

I am back on the couch downstairs, hiding in the basement. I keep reading Rebecca's texts. I want to ignore it all, but I can't. I stare at the stairs I grew up climbing. This basement used to be just cement and rafters. I remember making haunted houses down here. Then Dad remodeled it. He put in a bar that can seat nine people, a pool table, a big screen television, and a booth, like you see at a restaurant. There was plenty of room for all the parties and the people we had in and out over the years. Today I feel its emptiness. It hasn't been used in years. Dad could no longer do the stairs.

Even though it is the darkest place in the entire house it gives me the closest feeling to harmony available at this stage of my humanity.

I finally go up, to find Mom on a cleaning binge.

"What's going on?" I ask.

"William and Tracy are on their way."

She is in a frenzy, picking up blankets and pillows.

Same old Mom. There is a dying man in a hospital bed, in the middle of the living room, and she is worried about the tidiness of the house.

Dad yells out, "I have to *number two*."

Mom screams back at him, "Oh God, you're kidding?"

"Why would I kid about that? I have to take a shit."

"Oh Dick, you haven't shit since you've been home."

"I'm ready now, please Tweets."

"Geez and crackers, Dick, I can't believe you. William and Tracy are coming over."

"I can't help it, Tweets. I have to shit."

I run into the laundry room, grab the bed pan, and through the window see them walking toward the house. I run back to the bed, "Shit, they are on their way right now."

Mom shouts, "Oh Dick, can you wait?"

"Tweets, I have to shit. What don't you understand?"

I say, "Okay, let's just put it under him and leave it there till they leave. He will just have to wait."

Kate responds, "Good idea, let's do it."

Mom looks out the window and says, "God dammit, Richard, they're almost here."

Kate and I are holding him on his side as I yell, "Come on Mom, put it under him."

She screams, "I don't know which way it goes."

Kate and I look at the bizarre-shaped thing, and I finally yell, "Just stick it under there."

We roll him onto it just as the front door opens. Kate covers him up and says, "Okay Dad, we have company so you are going to just have to wait a bit."

He replies, "I'm not going to sit on this thing, it's too uncomfortable."

Mom whispers, "Richard, you need to be good,

William and Tracy are here."

They are frozen for about twelve seconds as they examine the bed and understand the man that lies on it, is dying.

William walks up to The Scene like he is on some kind of mission. Tracy follows, catches him, and they both grab the rails. William's knuckles bulge out as his fingers wrap the rail with empathy. "Hi Dick, how you feeling?"

Dad looks up, trying to see a face, "William, is that you?"

Tracy says, "Yeah, that's him, and I'm here too."

"I'm not in too good a shape."

William responds, "Yeah, I know, but I bet you're glad to be home?"

Dad replies, "William, it is wonderful, absolutely wonderful."

He then says, "Hey Molly, I have to go to the bathroom."

"Mom, Dad has to pee," I yell.

She doesn't respond. She is busy, ignoring the situation.

Tracy and William walk into the kitchen. Tracy says to Mom, "Dick has to go to the bathroom."

Mom, angry, walks toward The Scene, "Richard, they just got here."

He replies, "Tweedles, I can't take this thing under me anymore. It hurts too much."

I ask him, "Did you go?"

"No."

Kate and I roll him over, and Mom says, "Thank God, he just peed."

I walk into the kitchen. William is pouring Bailey's in his coffee.

I wash my hands, and notice the way William glares out at The Scene, his eyes glued to the bed.

It doesn't matter where you stand, you can't help but obsess over the unavoidable. Death is lurking. Dad, I'm sure, is embarrassed of his weakness. He can't fight it, and it humiliates him into silence. He plays it off, but still seeks pity with those he can. He is a smart man. He beat the system. He pretty much did what he wanted, all the time, without sacrifice. He worked hard in his younger years, but he never lived as a true family man. He had two different families, two different attempts, and he chose to live the same life, twice. He chose to be a Dick.

*

I can't sleep even though it's almost midnight. He is too needy for me to even try to close my eyes. I will just be disappointed when I have to open them to meet his next request.

"Molly, are you awake?" he asks.

"Yeah Dad."

He stutters a bit, "Will you pray with me so I can get better?"

A little surprised with his question, I ponder for a moment and reply, "Okay."

A few seconds go by and I fold my hands together as his voice mumbles, "Dear God—"

I can't make out what he is saying. It is gibberish to my ears, but it's okay because he is trying. He is seeking help.

Day 15

Kate has had the news on all day. There was an earthquake in Chile, and all they know is 147 people were found dead so far. The number has not increased since it first appeared on the screen, and it repeats about every three minutes.

"One hundred forty-seven dead," blurts from the box. It is the center of the room. I see it, I hear it, but what does it mean?

The house is full. Kate's kids, Ty and Samantha are here, as well as Curtis, Chloe and her husband, Nate.

Us girls sit at the table and play Hand and Foot.

I need a break, and run downstairs. The guys are playing pool. I tell Curtis, "Dad wanted me to pray with him, to get better."

Curtis sighs, "That sucks. That's just awful. Thank you for helping him. God, that sucks, poor Dad."

Acceptance is still not in Dad's realm. A prayer of hope should not be his concern; a plea for forgiveness is what he truly needs.

I'm back upstairs. We recall many family stories, and laughter is everywhere, but Dad does not agree with the entertainment.

He keeps asking, "When is everyone going to go home, so I can go to bed?"

I finally say, "Dad, you won't sleep anyway, even if everyone is gone. You are up all night."

With everyone here, I could shave a few hours off my shift. However, Dad once again gets his way, and the party ends early.

*

It is 11:52 p.m., and the third time I have been up since he supposedly went to sleep. This time, ice cream is his pleasure. I thought he was tired, but the night gets worse. I lie down, and he calls me up again, "Molly, Molly."

"What, Dad?"

"Come here."

"What?"

"Please come here."

My body moves upward and addresses the bed, "What Dad?"

"Go to bed, Skeeters."

"Go to bed? You just called me up here."

He screams out, "Come on Molly. Please let's go to sleep now."

Day 16

It's mid-morning when he asks, "Hey Molls, can you clean the wounds on my legs?"

The cancer is now popping up on his legs. Red bubbles yesterday, and today there are open wounds filled with a lime colored puss.

I try to clean the diseased flesh that is destroying his existence. He screams, "Jesus Christ, that hurts!"

Cleaning something that can't be healed is useless, but also essential. This makes no sense to me.

Mom, Kate, and I adjust his pillows. This time, it takes eight strategically positioned pillows to comfort his ache.

I am a lot like my dad. I always got whatever I wanted and I have always done exactly what I wanted. The reason I now know this is because lately it hasn't been like that. Confinement in this house has challenged my body and my mind.

The doorbell rings. I get up, and see the face through the window—*this can't be him.* I open the door, and he says, "Hi, I'm Gabe."

He is in his fifties, has a white Santa Claus beard, and seems a bit *red neck* for this situation. Kate's eyes widen as she shakes his hand. She is also taken aback by his appearance. He is wearing a big blue Eskimo parka, stonewashed jeans, and mountain boots.

This is the recommendation for home care from Heather?

He goes directly to The Scene, and says, "Hello Mr. Weasley, I'm Gabe. How are you feeling today?"

Dad responds, "How much is this going to cost?"

Mom snaps, "Richard, you are always concerned about the money, but we need help."

"Everything seems fine, Tweets. I don't know why we need home care?"

"The girls have to go home, and I can't do this alone. They have lives they have to get back to."

She turns and says to Gabe, "Let's sit down at the table and talk."

Gabe says, "I know you are worried about the money. I don't really think you need someone twenty-four hours, but I think someone at night would be your best bet. This way you have all day for him to tire you out and then you can get a good night's rest. I can tell you girls are on very minimal sleep."

Mom says, "Oh yeah, he is up all night. I don't think he sleeps. Does he Molly?"

"I don't think so," I respond.

"Probably not, he is scared of the darkness and if he closes his eyes he is scared that they may not open again," he says.

Mom and Gabe work out the details for overnight care.

Mom concludes the conversation saying, "Thank you so much. We will probably call you for Tuesday night."

Gabe walks up to the bed and says, "It was good to meet you Richard. I will see you soon. I look forward to our time together."

Kate shows him out, as Mom says, "I really like him."

Kate replies, "Yeah, very compassionate toward Dad."

Dad says, "Waste a' money, Ma."

Mom replies, "Oh Richard, don't worry about it."

Sunlight has disappeared when the door opens, and Claire walks through. Her face does not react to The Scene. Then again, her face has always had a somber look. Her hair is styled like something out of a zombie movie. Her bangs are up high and the sides are hair-sprayed out so they look like wings coming out of her head, like a vulture. She unties her baby blue trench coat, as she approaches him, "Hi Dad, how you doing?"

"Claire is that you?"

The door opens again, and Bridgett enters holding her baby, Hunter.

"There's my big boy," Claire says, leaving the bed to grab the baby. "Hunter is here. *Hello, Grandpa!*"

She puts the baby into Dad's view. Dad's hand slowly rises as he grabs one of the cute little blue sneakers. He jiggles the baby's foot and says, "Hi, Hunter boy."

Claire gives Bridgett the baby back and says, "Let me get my camera."

Claire takes tons of pictures with the baby and Dad, the baby and Bridgett, and even the baby and Kate. I can tell Mom is irritated. She finally says, "Richard, are you about ready for dinner?"

He replies, "Yeah, what are we having?"

"Meatloaf."

Bridgett says, "I put our dinner in the oven when we left, so we should go anyway."

Dad replies, "Yeah, I need to get to bed early tonight. I have a tee time in the morning."

"You have a tee time in the morning, with who?" Mom responds.

"Jackson."

Mom looks at us with a *what-the-heck* expression as she says, "Jackson was one of your Dad's best friends. He died about five years ago."

She asks, "Dick, who else are you playing with?"

He doesn't respond. She tries once more, "Richard, what time is your tee time?"

Still no answer, until he says, "Tweets, are you going to get my dinner?"

*

It's almost midnight, and this is the first time he has called me since I turned the television off at ten. I'm feeding him ice cream. He says, "When I'm done with this, we need to go to sleep. I have an early tee time."

"With who?"

"Jackson."

"Dad, where are you playing with Jackson?"

There is no response, as he swooshes the last spoonful of milky cold sugar in his mouth.

"Dad, what about your tee time? Who else is playing?"

"Skeets, will you rub my feet before we go to sleep?"

"Yeah Dad, but tell me about tomorrow?"

I start to massage his ankle.

"Dad, are you playing with Jackson in the morning?"

He doesn't reply.

"Dad, do you hear me?"

"Skeets, why are my feet burning up?"

"I don't know, Dad. Tell me about your tee time?"

"Are we going to go to sleep?"

"Yeah Dad, let's sleep."

"Okay, Skeets I'm tired."

Just grateful he wants to sleep, I lie down and curl up under the blanket, close my eyes, and drift off.

Day 17

Kate and I are holding him up, as Mom tries to maneuver a pillow underneath him. Compared to the nights before, there were minimal requests, but I'm still so tired that I can barely stand.

Mom says, "These sheets are disgusting. Look, these stains are from his tumor."

"All right, let's do the tumor, and then we'll do the sheets," I reply.

It is spongier today, and saturated. I notice a piece of metal protruding from the tissue. After a long delicate process, the metal of a staple glistens on the green rubber glove that covers my right index finger. Kate, Mom, and I all stare at the flimsy thing. It looks like it came from a stapler used in a kindergarten class.

Mom says, "Oh, must be from when they tried to cut the tumor out."

My stomach flips. I am clammy as I run to the kitchen. My hands straddle the sink, and my head falls in a woozy state. With my eyes closed, I am trying to get control of my insides. I open my eyes, and am taunted by an object in the sink. Flesh, oozing blood through the plastic, with numbers to represent the price, blasts my fragile pupils.

I scream, "Unbelievable!"

Mom shouts, "What is it?"

"Come here, look at this."

"What?"

"Just come over here. Please, Mom, please, come here."

"Okay, okay."

She still pauses before she walks over, saying, "Now, what is it, Molly?"

My finger extends in the sink. She sees the big white tag on the round steak reading $7.47. She looks up and her eyes pass the microwave.

She exclaims, "Geez and crackers, and it's 8:47, too!"

Does a similarity exist between Dad's blood, discolored and poisoned, and the blood of the round steak, pure and worthy of its maker? The tag on this piece of meat reads $7.47, but the value is priceless. Value is important when it comes to love and forgiveness. My father is a man who valued himself, and cared little for those who loved him. He didn't sacrifice, but believes others should sacrifice for him. These digits did not conspire to occur together. The time may be 8:47, but more important, is the circumstance. Identifying sin, as sin, is important when admitting to unrighteousness, but it is not the last assessment. Repentance of transgressions, changes the moment of captivity to everlasting life. Without forgiveness, his days of anguish will linger.

Dad should be well situated after the morning we've had. Kate and I are trying to get comfortable in our seats, knowing we will be in them the rest of the day. Mom feeds Dad breakfast. She looks like *shit* – tired, depressed, and old.

He says to Mom, "Just pull the plug."

"Pull the plug? There is no plug," she says.

"What about the machine back there?"

"It's your oxygen tank."

"Pull the plug," he says.

Kate explains to him, "You are not on life support, Dad. You're not even on the oxygen. There is no machine keeping you alive."

"Oh," he sighs. "Can I have a cookie?"

Mom scurries out to play Hand and Foot at the neighbor's house. Kate and I tend to Dad.

The doorbell rings. I look through the window to see another familiar face. Nothing has changed since I was a kid; friends are still always in and out of the house. Lynn embraces me. She says, "I'm meeting Leslie here. I told her I wanted to help out."

My achy body nestles into hers. Her arms are around me, but her head has turned to Dad. She is still as she ingests The Scene. She reacts to her vision, her arms leave me, and she moves toward him. "Hi Dick, how are you doing, now that you're home?"

Dad replies, "Lynn, is that you? Where is the big guy?"

He is referring to her husband, Zack. Dad and Zack played a lot of golf through the years. They spent many days together.

Kate leisurely stretches and sits upright from a nap.

"Lynn this is my sister, Kate."

Kate puts her feet on the floor, "Hi, Lynn, it's nice to meet you."

"Oh please don't get up, I'm sure you guys are exhausted. Please relax."

The doorbell chimes again. Lynn says, "That must be Leslie."

I reply, "No, it's Bud."

Bud was Dad's boss and the owner of the golf course. He is about a quarter of the way through the door when his eyes stick to The Scene.

"Here is the number your mother asked for," he says,

as his hand shoves a piece of paper into my hand. Bud's focus is on the man in the bed. He walks to The Scene, and says, "Hi Dick."

Dad replies, "Hi Bud, I'm sorry, but I'm a bit under the weather."

"I know, and I'm sorry to hear. I gave Molly a phone number of a good lady. Her name is Dee, and she helped my mom when she was in hospice. Hopefully, she can help you too."

Dad replies, "That would be nice."

Bud takes Dad's hand and says, "I have to go, but you take care, okay."

"I'll try my best, Bud. Thanks for stopping by."

Bud pauses at the door.

Frozen in a moment of truth, he conceives the reality of what is before him – a friend who suffers today and dies tomorrow.

*

All the visitors have left, and Mom is still gone. Kate is on her couch and I sit in Mom's chair. I am looking down on her side table, full of papers and things. There is a lottery ticket with the mega number 47. To the right, is a list of home care agencies, their phone numbers all beginning with 847. The number that Bud gave me lies on top, and of course, the first three digits are 477.

When I first started keeping track of my score, my goal was to shoot 47 for nine holes. Soon enough, I was scoring 48 to 52, depending on a good or bad day. The goal to shoot 47 became the goal of the summer, and the next, and then finally, it almost happened. I just finished the sixth hole, it was pushing dark, and drizzling. If I played the next hole it would put me farthest from the house, but I was in the middle of my best round ever and I had to finish. The thunder began to roll, but I didn't care. I sprinted to the next tee box, put the ball on the tee and swung – another great shot. I skipped down the mound and onto the fairway. The lightening crackled, as I hit my second shot about eight feet from the pin. I missed the putt, but I still made par. Only two holes away from finishing, even if I bogeyed out, I would still shoot 42, which was way below my goal. However, the rain got heavier, and turned to hail. The thunder was loud and the wind howling. I needed to get home.

I ran as fast as I could, with my golf bag banging on my short body and the club heads beating against my neck. I held my shoulder strap tight, trying to resist the bag's movement. Puddles were forming. I focused on my feet splashing through the grass. It was coming down so hard that I couldn't see in front of me as I approached our street.

I got to the garage, and took my bag off of my shoulders. I sat on the doorstep to catch my breath, and wiped my eyes with a towel. I took off my shoes and socks, got up, and walked back to the edge of the garage where I wrung out my socks. I grabbed a soda from the fridge before walking into the house. Mom was making dinner and Dad was in his chair. Mom said, "Oh Molls, you are soaking wet."

"I know. I'm going to change."

I walked into the living room, "Hey Dad, I got a question."

"Okay, Skeets."

"What happens if you are playing a round and can't finish because it starts to storm?"

"Well the pros would mark their ball where it was last hit and then go back out and start from that spot when the rain lets up."

"And their score would count for the first holes, even if they didn't finish the same day?"

"Yeah Skeets, as long as they finish when the storm lets up and they start play exactly from where they stopped."

"Okay, good. So I can go back out tomorrow and finish, because I only had two holes left and I had the best score I have ever had so far."

"Who were you playing with?"

"No one. I was by myself."

"You were by yourself? That's just practice, it doesn't really count. Your score doesn't count unless you have someone playing with you."

"But I played really good – my best round ever."

"Well Skeets, normally you need at least one other person playing with you for it to count."

I never did go back out and finish the round.

I am reclined, with my back to the front door, when Mom walks in. She whispers to herself, "Everyone is asleep, good."

Dad's voice sounds pathetic, "I'm awake, Tweets."

Mom says, "Oh Richard, you need to rest."

I sluggishly move my muscles, and say, "Bud was here. He gave me a number for a home care lady."

Mom walks up to the bed and asks Dad, "Dick, did you see Bud?"

"Yeah, Tweets. I have to pee."

"Okay, Richard."

She gets him ready to pee as she asks him, "So what did you and Bud talk about?"

"Nothin' Tweets. He just came by to say hi."

"That's all he said to you, was *hi*?"

"He knows I'm under the weather, Tweets. Everyone who comes here knows I'm not feeling well. Now, when are we going to eat dinner? I'm hungry, Tweets."

"Geez and crackers, you are a piece of work, Dick Weasley. A piece of work."

I turn on the television to relieve the tension. Kate and I are relaxed and almost lost from the situation until Mom says, "Dinner is ready."

I walk to the table with a plate of beef stroganoff. The substance on the plate slides suddenly, but my hand is able to calm the rattled food, and only a few noodles fall to the floor. I kneel down to pick up the evidence, as Mom and Kate tend to their plates. This is easy, compared to the last time I recall this happening, about 20 years ago.

I was just a kid and the fact that the carpet was only a few hours old didn't trigger my hand to slip, but Mom thought differently. It was spaghetti, and it was more than just a few noodles. I'm not sure what happened, but on the way from the kitchen to the living room, my marinara and meatballs took a terrible fall. I remember Mom yelling at me so bad that I got on my bike to run away.

*

It's 1:28 a.m. and his voice is constant, with an annoying, unintelligible mumble. I know I should say something to him, but can't figure out what.

His bag is heavy, as I tread with him down these dreary fairways. However, this difficult match might lead to a night without disturbance, a night of peace. Peace would be my greatest victory, but since he doesn't have any within himself, he sure has none to share with me.

Day 18

"Molly I have to pee. It's morning, Skeeters, get up."

"Okay, Dad."

I unwrap the blanket from my body and rise to another gloomy day.

Eight nights in a row I have constantly tended to his every call, but eight is enough. Tonight I will finally get silence.

Mom's voice is soft, as she walks down the hallway. She is on the phone and says to whomever, "Maybe due to his life, he is suffering."

If Mom had to deal with his unruly life, then why does she have to grieve about the way he leaves?

The door opens and Heather says, "Good morning."

She approaches The Scene, "Hi Richard."

He doesn't respond.

"How are you feeling today?"

"Tired, and I'm hungry. I haven't had my breakfast yet."

"Oh Richard, I will start it right now. Geez and crackers, you just woke up."

His eyes seem bluer than normal.

Heather says, "You have great eyes."

He doesn't respond.

Heather goes to the fridge and pulls out a box. She put it in there the first day, but today explains its importance. She describes the purpose of each medicine and when to use them, "Normally when we begin this, the dying process has started. You may not use it for a while, but if the symptoms occur use it immediately."

Mom says, "There's no morphine in there, right? 'Cause he can't have that."

"No, there is not. They are sedatives, but nothing like morphine, and when you do use it you will start off with the lowest dose. If he begins to get agitated or upset in any way give him a dose of each drop."

*

Kate leaves soon and then it will be just Mom, Dad, and me.

I'm scared in my bones that this is going to get worse. I'm getting off the kiddy ride and getting on the roller coaster. The last time I was on a roller coaster my marriage ended. A picture was taken as we fell from the sky. My husband looked frightened, with his head hidden in his hands, as I smiled big at the world. How could one be so miserable, and one be so happy, at the exact same time? It was the ride on that coaster that concluded our commitment once and for all. It was the best ride of my life.

Babe and Henry arrive to take Kate to the airport.

Mom asks Dad, "Are you gonna' miss Kate?"

Dad stutters, "Without a doubt."

Kate leans in to Dad, "I love you Dad. Talk to God, okay?"

"Okay. I love you, Katie."

Kate departs but we remain, baffled and unsure of the next week, day, or even moment to come.

I never understood how God could exist, but I find myself opening up to the idea. Confusion is a feeling that won't leave me. Fear isn't as heavy today, but anger is strong.

Mom is preoccupied easily. She does this subconsciously, to avoid the situation at hand. This is why we need help. She can't be alone with him, which is why I am here, and probably will be for a while. I ask Mom, "Do you think now that Kate is gone, Claire will come out?"

"I don't think so, Molls. When Dad was in the hospital she told me she went through this with her mom and she wasn't going to go through it again."

Well, she isn't. I am.

There are no visitors today. It has been quiet, and I feel like a kid again—trapped in the house, with the two of them, in the dead of winter.

Time is reflection. I am beginning to understand the purpose of the bed. He suffers physical pain, but he also suffers mentally, remembering his life, and the sins he ignored.

Mom says to Dad, "Now Richard, Gabe is going to be here soon."

No response.

He is not happy about what is going to take place. However, I couldn't be more thrilled.

Gabe arrives, and within seconds Mom and I are off to bed. With Kate gone, I get my room back. The darkness and the silence are inviting. The bed swallows my body and massages it without interruption throughout the night.

Day 19

Gabe whispers, "Tweedy."

My eyes open, it seems as though I've been asleep for hours, but it is still dark out. I open the door and walk down the hall. I squint at the shimmer of his wavy, silver hair on the white of the pillow, illuminated by the doorbell light.

Mom and Gabe are at the bed. Mom notices me and says, "Can you believe it? First time he's peed."

"What time is it?" I ask.

Gabe responds, "Five-thirty. Yeah, he was quiet most the night. I got up twice to give him a sip of soda."

Anger boils in my blood – he kept me up for eight nights straight and now he barely needed anything last night.

I curl up in a ball, and let the bed capture me again.

It's almost 9:30 when I approach his side. He says, "Molly, help me get out of this bed."

"Dad, you are not going to get out of the bed."

I tend to his wounds.

Mom had to run out, and I sit a few feet from his

deathbed, in silence. I can't help but watch him. I can see he is thinking.

Until he assimilates his past, present, and most important, his future, the burning will only increase. If the flames get too big, will the gates of Hell engulf him? He is terrified and I know I need to talk to him, but I don't know how.

"Hey Molls, help me get into the chair."

"I can't Dad, you're too heavy."

"Go get Mom, she can help."

"Dad, you can't get out of the bed, you are too weak. You have to understand. Do you understand?"

"But Skeets, if you just move the chair over here, I will slide in."

"It's not that easy, I'm sorry Dad, but you are not getting out of the bed."

Leslie walks in, "How we doin' today?"

Her timing is always perfect.

She walks up to Dad. "Hi Dick, how you feelin' today?"

"It would be nice if I could sit in my chair, but Molly won't help me get out of the bed."

"Unfortunately, Molly can't help you out of the bed. You have to stay in the bed. I'm so sorry, but your time here is ending, and in order for you to move on and get out of the bed, you have to wait until it's your time. God will let you know when he is ready for you to get out of the bed."

"But I need to get out now. I'm in pain, and my feet are on fire. I need to move around."

"I know, Dick. We will move you a bit, and get you

repositioned, but that's all we can do. You have to talk to God. You may not be ready to see Him yet, but you have to talk to Him. Let Him know you are ready and He will take you."

"Skeets, my crack hurts again. Can you stick a pillow under there?"

"Okay, Dad."

Leslie maneuvers him best she can, as I shove the pillow under him. He screams, "Ouch! God damn that hurts."

"Sorry, Dick. Sorry. We are just trying to get you comfortable."

"Let's clean his tumor," I say to Leslie.

With a flashlight, we examine the open wound under his arm. There is no specific mass, just a hole of raw tissue. This is the pit where the venom was born. A cutout shape creeps out over half his right breast and into the areola, with plans to devour his nipple.

The seeping poison takes over his body, but his tarnished soul has a chance to be renewed. We, the close ones, recognize Dad's downfall, but can't comprehend his denial. Reluctant to accept, he intensifies his parting. Goodbye is not something he will say. Endearment is not something he will show. He must understand his life, his death, and his fate before the disease consumes his entire core. Today he feels sorry for himself, so he will not die today. Tomorrow gives him another opportunity. He can, like all the days before, soak in self-pity or he can emerge from it and allow forgiveness to purify the shame that burdens him.

A friend Mom used to work with stops by. She walks in and her eyes glue to The Scene. Excitement covers Mom's face as she rejoins with her pal. They sit on the couch and talk about the bank. Thirty minutes go by, and still not a word about Dad. Mom loves the attention of an outsider who is unfamiliar with the situation.

Dad is in his spot, Mom is preoccupied with something, and I stare at the television.

After an hour of indulgent conversation, Mom tells her friend how Dad ended up eight feet away in a hospital bed. She gets up and walks toward the silver rail.

"Richard, Michelle is here," she says.

Michelle comes to the bed and says, "Hi, Dick."

Dad replies, "Hi Michelle. Where's your cocktail?"

"Oh, not tonight, have to wait for Mexico."

Dad proceeds to ask her about her husband and her golf game.

Michelle was not captured by the scene, like most before her, but as she walks out the door, she takes a quick final glance at the picture of death, or of life, to hold in her mind.

*

Mom and I are both asleep when the doorbell rings.

"Come on in," I yell from the couch.

Gabe enters and says, "Hi, how is Mr. Richard tonight?"

I reply, "He is all yours, 'cause I'm going to bed."

Mom says, "Me too."

She leisurely gets out of her chair and says, "Hi Gabe, how are you?"

"I'm good, Tweedy. You girls look exhausted. Has Richard been keeping you on your toes?"

"He can be a piece of work sometimes, Gabe. Let me tell you, I lived with this man for thirty-five years, and yes,

I'm very tired."

She approaches the bed, leans in and kisses Dad, "Goodnight, Richard."

"Goodnight, Tweets."

I lean in and kiss his cheek, "Night Dad, I love you."

"Love you too, Skeets."

Day 20

The soda bubbles, as I put the glass up to my mouth. Fizzes shoot up and tickle my nose. I take a sip.

Mom says, "Gabe said Dad was up all night."

"Oh, really? What happened?"

"He said they talked about God."

"They did? Like what, what did he say?"

"I don't know, but he didn't sleep at all, he kept Gabe up all night."

I walk over to The Scene, "Did you and Gabe talk last night?"

"Yeah, we talked a little bit."

"What did you talk about?"

"I need more pop, Skeets."

"Tell me what Gabe said to you."

"Please Molls, my pop."

"No, Dad. Not until you tell me what you talked to Gabe about."

"I don't remember, Skeets."

"Yes you do, Dad. You talked about God. Now tell me about it."

"He talked about God, I just listened. Now, I'm begging you to please get me some pop."

Mom walks up, "Here is your pop, Richard."

She puts the straw in his mouth, "Very naughty, a very naughty man you are. Did you listen to what Gabe said?"

Dad is still sucking the straw.

"Richard, Richard, I'm asking you a question. Do you know what Gabe said?"

"Why are you such a donkey nuts?" he yells.

The doorbell rings and Amy enters, "Morning."

Mom replies, "Morning, Amy. He's all yours."

I take the opportunity to run downstairs.

When I return, Mom is at The Scene telling Amy, in her saddest voice, "I don't know what I'm going to do when Molly goes back."

Amy walks by me with the blue tub, "When do you have to go back, Molly?"

"I really don't know yet."

Mom says, "Molly hasn't been out of the house in days."

"Eleven to be exact," I comment.

Amy says, "You need to get out. I'm going to call and see if I can get you a nurse for tomorrow."

We are here meeting his every need. But he never would do the same for us. We hardly ever spent time as a family. I blamed Mom for working, but it was him the whole time. I've always wondered why Dad didn't come with us to Disney World. It was a big family trip, and he just didn't come. Grandma came in his place, and I never understood why. I see now, it was the middle of summer, golf season.

At 10:24 a.m. he asks, "Molly, how am I going to get out of the bed?"

Like a teacher to a student, I explain, "Dad, the only way you are going to get out of this bed is to accept whatever it is you need to accept, and then you will go to Heaven and you will be able to do whatever you want: walk, run, golf, you name it."

No response.

I start again, "Do you hear what I am saying?"

In a wimpy, but clear voice, he replies, "Yes."

Dad and I doze, while Mom fusses around the house. A couple of hours later the doorbell rings and an Asian woman with a short haircut, wearing scrubs, walks in. This was the lady Bud referred for home care. Mom made an appointment with her to see about getting more help when I leave. I'm in a bit of a mood and don't care to join them at the table, so I sit in my chair and watch. Mom somehow turns the conversation to when she was let go from her job.

When I was growing up, she always talked about work. It's so familiar, as though I'm a child again, reliving certain moments through my senses.

The woman goes over to the bed, "Hi Mr. Weasley, I'm Dee."

She starts moving him and rolling him around like he is nothing. He is not pleased with her tactic, and yells at her to stop. She continues, so he shouts out, "Molly!"

"What is it Dad?"

"I'm ready to accept the Big Guy."

"You are?"

"I can't take girls roughing me around like this."

"Well then, accept it because this is what you have to deal with if you don't."

Dee says to me, "I'm free tonight, if you want to get out. I could do a 12-hour shift, so you could sleep through the night."

Mom cancels Gabe for the night, and we take Dee up on her offer.

She barely gets out of the door, and Dad hollers, "I don't want her coming back."

"Molly hasn't been out of this house in days. You will be fine."

Through the window I see Dee drive onto the main street. Another car pulls in.

"Eddie and Shelly are here," I exclaim.

The more people in the house, the lighter the atmosphere.

Shelly opens the door and says, "How's my little Weasel doing?"

Eddie stands 6'4", is broad shouldered, and has slicked-back gray hair that starts high on his forehead. He is a quiet man, mostly because ninety percent of the time his mouth is preoccupied with a stogie.

His eyes meet The Scene.

Shelly approaches the bed and says again, "How's my little Weasel?"

"Shells, is that you?"

"Yeah, and Eddie is with me."

"Hi Dick. How are you feeling?"

"Big Eds, is that you?"

"It's me, Weasel."

He reaches the bed's side.

Misery glazes Dad's eyes, even as he greets his friend. Eddie continues, "How does it feel to be home, Dick?"

"Eds, I can't tell you how great it is. It's wonderful, just wonderful."

"I bet it is. This is a nice set up you got."

"You can say that again, Big Eds."

We tell them we are now free for the evening, and they immediately invite us over.

Mom says, "I really like Dee, I think she will be good."

Dad yells, "I would prefer she not come back."

"She's coming. Mom and I need to get out!" I shout.

Mom grabs the soda from my hand, walks toward Dad, and in a stern voice says, "Richard, now you be good to Dee."

Mom stares at him, as he looks at the soda in her hand. She waits for some response.

"Come on Tweets, give me my pop. I'm thirsty," he cries.

"Did you hear me Dick? I mean it, you better be nice to her."

He snaps back, "I'm gonna' pinch her titty."

We all laugh.

"Richard, you wouldn't do that, would you?" Shelly replies.

*

Mom and I are in the office, and she types in a password on her computer, M-O-L-L-Y. Through the window I see Leslie pull up and I hurry to greet her. Soon we are all standing around the bed arguing with Dad about why he can't have a scooter. Leslie says, "Dick, right now, you have to wait, and when the Lord is ready, you will be with him. While you wait, pray for forgiveness. You need to put your faith in the Lord."

Dad questions himself, 'Does God want my soul back after I have dirtied it?' He is embarrassed to even approach the Lord, so he lies in agonizing pain, and slithers away in his own regret. His sins haunt him and strengthen his will to overcome death. He needs to accept himself. Once he knows he is forgiven, he can reach his destiny.

*

I have been trapped in the house, but as we pull out of the garage my thoughts are still with him, and I am worried.

Dee was a bit rough with him. What if she hurts him, or what if he dies while we are away? I can't allow that to happen. I need to be there. I was never of significance to him, but today he is my whole existence.

Day 21

Heather is at his side when I emerge from my room, she says to Mom, "My twenty-five year old thinks so too."

"You have a twenty-five year old? How old are you?" I ask, as I drop onto the couch to watch her prepare his day.

"Forty-seven."

"Forty-seven, how can you be forty-seven?" I reply.

"You may not think so, but I am."

"Of course you are! Why wouldn't you be?"

"Oh my God, forty-seven? I can't believe it," Mom says.

I shake my head, "How ridiculous."

Mom explains the coincidental occurrences of the two stupid digits to Heather.

The one who nurses him into death and helps him comfortably leave the Earth was born forty-seven years ago. A year is an amount of time, and a distance in a life. She is connected; chosen to aid his diseased heart. She doesn't realize it, but I do. Many forces surround The Scene wanting Dad to regain his righteousness.

After a shower, I run up the stairs and ask Mom, "Do you have another hair dryer I can just keep downstairs?"

"Yeah, hold on."

I run back downstairs with the mini blue hair dryer, but within seconds I see a flame out of the corner of my eye, and realize it is on fire. I unplug it and throw it in the sink, "Unbelievable, Mom."

I finish getting ready the best I can, walk back up-stairs, and throw the broken dryer in the garbage.

Mom and I put our coats on, but Dad is not pleased, "Where are you going to eat?"

"The Noodle Garden," Mom says.

"That's too much money for lunch. You should stay here and take care of me."

"We have to get out Dick. We are just going to lunch. We'll be back in a couple hours."

"You girls have fun. We'll be fine, right Dick?" Heather says.

As we pull out of the driveway, I point to the screen on the dash, "It's 1:47."

"Oh my God," Mom responds.

Another adventure of liberty begins.

The topic of the conversation is how Dad is a true asshole, along with Aunt Judy yelling at the waitress.

"Is that English you're speaking, because I can't understand you," she blurts out, and it echoes off the walls.

Aunt Judy was the one with all the backbone, Dad never an ounce. 'Feel sorry for me' is his way out, but that's not good enough this time. Judgment day has come.

The house is filled with voices as we walk in from lunch. Lynn, with her husband Zack and another couple, David and Kitty are at The Scene.

David and Kitty used to live in the neighborhood; I grew up with them. We spent many nights on their deck. In fact, I got engaged on their deck, with Lynn and Zack there too. Mom and Kitty were best friends; when they moved, it was hard on her.

It's so strange to see them here, next to Dad's deathbed.

We all sit around, and Dad takes in the familiar voices.

He says, "Hey Ma, have David and Zack wheel me to the side of the house."

Mom asks, "What? What are you talking about?"

"Wheel me to the side of the house, Tweets. Please, the guys can help."

"Why, why do want to do that?"

He ignores her question at first, but soon murmurs, "I have to pee."

Mom prepares for the task; David and Zack flee to the garage. Dad looks up at Mom and with fury whines, "Dammit, Tweets. That's why I wanted you to have them wheel me to the side of the house, so I could pee in private."

"Oh Richard, that makes no sense."

The guys come back in to say goodbye.

New fans stand on the sidelines, and once again, The Scene captivates them, leaving an indelible vision of their friend's passing.

Mom and I finally relax in our chairs, hoping he permits us rest.

Next, Curtis and Chloe walk through the door.

"How's Pops doing today?" Curtis says as he walks up to the bed.

"I don't feel like I'm getting any better."

"Well, are you eating? We brought you some fish fry."

Dad says, "Oh, that sounds good."

I get him a plate, because I know we will hear about it if he does not have it in front of him soon. His appetite contradicts his affliction.

I also indulge in the fish fry I grew up on.

Midwest mentality comes out in my mother as she starts to justify my divorce to everyone. She announces, "Molly says Trent drank a lot and it really bothered her. I didn't realize he drank that much, but she says it was too much."

Continuously, she advocates the termination of my marriage. She now has a legitimate reason to spread all over the land. She thinks this justification will bring acceptance of me, and more importantly her.

Chloe, Curtis, Mom, and I roll him, trying to get his pillows situated because it will be a while before there is someone here to help us again.

*

The house is empty. I had a nice break the last few nights, away in my own bed, in my own room. Tonight I lie again beside the brown metal frame. Mom, amused by her program and well rested, stays with me for almost half the night.

It's 2:39 a.m., as I stare at the doorbell light waiting for him to finish his business.

"Dad, please, go to sleep now, okay?"

"Yeah Skeets, but I need a sip of pop first."

I'm walking to the kitchen, and he yells, "And some ice cream too, Skeets."

"Oh Dad, ice cream, really?"

My head finally sinks into the pillow. However, the doorbell light is battling with my pupils and I lie awake.

It was my senior year of high school, and I was coming home from school one afternoon in my little red Chevy. As I turned onto the street where the golf course is, I recognized Dad and his friends. David, Don, and Dad were walking up to the 11th green. I pulled over and ran up to the green and yelled, "Hey Dad!"

He waved and yelled back, "Hi Skeets, your mom is at Fall Diddley with the girls."

Don was knelt down on the green reading his putt. It was a ridiculously long putt, about forty feet. He looked over at me and said, "Get your clubs and join us."

"I can't, I have to get ready and go to work. Bye guys."

I darted down the hill and got back into my car.

As I always did back then, I ran halfway down the stairs, stopped and yelled, 'Geronimo!' as I leaped to the bottom, landing on both feet. I walked into the bathroom, opened the shower door, turned the handle, and then took off my clothes. I entered the steam and inhaled the smell of the metallic water.

I closed my eyes and was almost in a dream, when there was the sound of footsteps pounding down the stairs. I turned the water off, opened the shower door, and grabbed the towel. A loud knock forced me to jump. Dad's voice was scratchy and crackled, "Molly, Molly."

"Dad?"

"Molls, Don's dead, I have to go to the hospital."

"What, what do you mean?"

"Don's dead. I have to go."

"What? Wait, wait a minute."

"I have to go, David is waiting."

"Dad? Dad?"

I opened the door, walked out with the towel around me, picking up speed, and sprinted to the top of the stairs. Dad was not in sight, and the street was empty.

The house was dark when I pulled in the driveway after work. "Oh please be home, don't tell me you guys are out."

I got out of the car and walked toward the door. I could see a head through the glass, illuminated by the doorbell light. My heart was pounding.

Mom said, "Hi Molls, how was work?"

"Okay. Why are you sitting in the dark with that stupid light? Why can't we get rid of that thing?"

"What thing?"

"The doorbell light, I hate that thing."

"Oh Molly, I don't think we can get rid of it."

"Well, why are you sitting in the dark?"

"You know what happened to Don? He died. He was with your dad."

"I know, I know, I saw him."

"You did? When?"

"Coming home from school. I talked to him on eleven. He had a long putt."

Mom, hesitant, said, "He made that putt. Dad said the ball fell in the hole and Don fell to the ground."

Don's death must have suffocated Dad's thoughts. I didn't

recognize it then as much as I do now. He never talked about Don and he was always quiet if Don was mentioned. We never talked about what happened after I ran down the hill and got in my car. I'm sure Dad never stood on the 11th green again without worry of the unknown.

"Skeets, hey Skeets."

My eyes open, but I don't respond.

"Molly, Molls, please answer me."

"Fine Dad, but you better really need whatever it is you are going to ask me for."

"Okay Skeets, I promise."

"All right. What is it Dad?"

"Skeets, will you pray with me?"

My head turns toward him, "What?"

"Will you pray with me?"

"Yeah, Dad. Of course."

"Our Father, who art in Heaven," he begins.

I join in. Every word rolls off my tongue as though I was in the seventh grade again. In the darkest hour of the night I sit, detached, reciting the Lord's Prayer with my stricken father.

Day 22

His voice and the light hit me at the same instant, "Molly, is your mom up? Where's Mom?"

I ignore his plea.

A new day, a new tactic: I'm in charge and I'll respond on my terms.

"Molly, come on, get up, it's morning. We need to get up."

"All right, Dad. It's only 6:30. We need to try to sleep a little longer."

"Can I have an orange first?"

How many oranges will I feed him, or bowls of ice cream will he eat? This waiting is long and thick.

I stand at the counter, peeling his orange, taking in The Scene.

I'm back at the bed and after a long process of chewing, he says, "Thanks Skeets, that's the best orange I've ever had."

"Good Dad. Glad to hear. Now, I have to go to the bathroom. I will be back in a bit. Please do not wake up Mom."

I can barely walk down the stairs. I reach the bottom, and the couch invites me for a rest.

Footsteps from above awaken me.

"Shit, I fell asleep," I mutter.

It's almost 9:30 a.m., when I sprint up the stairs.

Mom asks me, "You want a bagel?"

"Yeah, what's going on?"

"He's on a roll already. He's hungry and wants to take a shower."

"Great," I say.

I turn around and head to The Scene, "Hi Dad."

"Molly, can you help me get out of the bed?"

"Dad, you are not getting out of the bed, remember?"

"What about my shower?"

"You don't take a shower anymore."

He yells, "I'm supposed to lay here and die?"

I respond, equally as angry, "You don't have to. You can pray and let go. I told you the only way out of the bed is Heaven."

His eyes widen, but he quickly dismisses the thought and says, "I want milk with my bagel."

As soon as the conversation interrupts his calmness, he must flee. Confrontation is something he does not do. The Lord does not want the soul of a coward. For another day peace will not exist, but will be prayed for.

*

I hear voices as I walk up from an easing shower. Grandma's giggly voice screeches, "There's my girl. How's Grandma's sweetheart."

Her arms gather my weary frame.

Aunt Susan rises from her chair with open arms, "How you holding up, kiddo?"

"Tired, just tired," I reply.

Mom explains, "He keeps her up all night, but when we have home care he's fine."

Aunt Susan says, "He wants to spend time with you."

"Yeah, but he doesn't say anything to me," I whisper.

Mom says, "Let's play cards."

Grandma tends to his need while we begin. A couple cookies and a lot of sips of pop later, Grandma sits back down, "Boy, he sure does like his soda."

We engross ourselves in the game, without worry for a moment.

Silence breaks too soon as he yells out, "When we gonna' eat lunch?"

Grandma peeps back, "You still hungry? You want Grandma to get you the frosty?"

"Yeah." he sighs.

The doorbell rings, and I respond, going to the door. Bonnie and Chester, friends from the playground we live upon, are waiting outside. The cold is sharp on my skin as I open the door. The smiles they show through the window change as they come through the doorway.

The entrance again brings shock to the uninitiated.

They each carry a box; I take Chester's and Mom helps Bonnie.

Bonnie says, "I brought you dinner."

"Dinner? This looks like a Thanksgiving feast," I say.

Chester approaches The Scene, "Hi Weasel."

"Is that Chester? Hi Chester."

"We wanted to come by and say hi. I'm sure you're happy to be home."

"You can say that again."

Mom asks, "What's that?"

Chester says, "I asked him if he is glad to be home."

Dad yells out, "You can say that again."

Bonnie reaches The Scene and says, "And I'm sure the food is better here, right Dick?"

Dad's eyes widen, as he says, "You can say that again."

Laughing, Chester gets a chair and sits next to Dad.

They talk about golf and the course.

I wonder what their thoughts really are. Dad and I haven't had many conversations, except for when he wants to get out of the bed. He lies close to me all day, but we never have a casual chat.

"We're gonna' go now Dick," Grandma says and kisses him sweetly.

She then leans into Chester and whispers, "Now, you keep talking to him, he likes your company."

All the holes are different and all the days are tough, but the support of the beloved fan inspires even the weakest competitor. This final round he plays is not easy for a spectator to watch. He is frail and suffering. However, he knows even at his worst, a full gallery is better than an empty one. To finish the last hole and walk off the green without anyone to run to, can be the loneliest moment.

By the time I was sixteen, I had played in many junior golf tournaments. I had already won and placed many times, and had many horrible rounds as well. However, out of all of them, a particular event stands out. Mom had to work, so she couldn't go. Dad was busy too – he had a tee time that couldn't be missed. Yet, I'm sure it was booked way after Mom paid my entry fee for the tournament.

I pulled into the parking lot of the country club, as the clock on the car radio turned 12:25. I quickly got out of the car, opened the trunk, and grabbed my clubs.

"Molly Weasley, last call for Molly Weasley," echoed from a megaphone. I saw the first tee and the man with the megaphone right away. I screamed, "I'm coming! I'm here! Wait!"

Everyone was looking at me approaching the tee box. The man said, "That was your last call. You exceeded your five minute warning and you will be assessed a two stroke penalty on this hole. So your tee shot will be your third shot."

I'm out of breath as I reply, "What? You've got to be kidding?"

"No, I'm not. You are up, and we are now behind. Please hit your tee shot."

I proceeded to hit a great drive and started out with a par, but a double bogey was my score, due to a freeway detour I didn't understand.

At the end of eighteen holes I was tied for the lead, and began a playoff with another girl. We started on the first tee, again. We both hit a perfect drive, not even feet apart. I was first to hit my second shot. I hit a five iron about eight feet from the pin. The other girl hit her ball to the right of the green, into a bunker. She proceeded to hit a superb shot out of the trap, but it still was not as close as my second shot. She missed her par putt, and I made my birdie putt. However, nobody cared. She had about five people surrounding her as she walked off the green in second place. I sauntered back to the scoreboard, alone, as dusk came over the sky. I followed her and her gallery into the clubhouse as though I was the one who lost the event. The trophy was handed to me, but somehow I received the least applause.

"We better get going, Chester," Bonnie says, as she gets up and approaches The Scene.

Chester says to Dad, "Well Dick, we have to go. You hang in there. We'll see you soon."

Dad replies, "Okay Chester, thanks for stopping by. Goodbye, Bonnie."

She softly tells him, "Dick, you keep eating Tweedy's good meals and you will feel better."

"I do already," he hollers out.

"It was great seeing you. I'm so glad you came by. And thanks for the food. You didn't have to do that. That's a lot of food," Mom's voice quakes as she hugs Bonnie.

The four of us stand in the foyer and say goodbye. Chester gazes one last time at the brown metal frame and sees the friend that it holds.

I go into Mom's office and sit down at her desk. I get on the Internet and search for flights. Mom's footsteps are heavy; she enters the room, and says, "Here is my credit card."

She sets it on the desk. I respond, "I found a flight for Friday, but I'm not sure I'm ready yet."

"You need to go back and get a job, before you lose your place."

The phone rings, and she runs out. I get to the payment screen for the ticket. I grab the credit card from the edge of the desk. Ready to type in the number, I look down and just laugh.

I can't do it. I can't leave until it's over.

I clear the screen, and get up. "Mom, Mom!" I shout.

"What? I'm on the phone," she yells back.

I walk through the living room, handing her the card.

"Your credit card begins and ends with 4-7."

I head to my dungeon.

My eyes are heavy and my face is pale in the mirror. Inhaling the herb calms me. I call the friend that is watching my dogs in California, tell him that I cannot come back as planned, and he agrees to continue his duty.

I hang up the phone and my knees give out. I fall against the wall and to the floor. Tears fill my eyes and stream like nothing I can recall. Emotionally, I have collapsed. I feel unprepared for the days to come.

*

It's almost dark. I am uncomfortable and bleary, but fixed to The Scene.

"Molly, did Mom start dinner?"

"Yeah Dad, Bonnie brought dinner, we are going to eat soon."

"Maybe, I should have a cookie while we wait."

"Okay, Dad."

Unhurried, I get out of the chair and make my way to the kitchen. It's like I am in the shell of a turtle, burdened and weighed down. I meet his demand. My actions are empty and robotic.

Dad's time in the world was always more important than anyone else's. He purposely made waiting a hobby. Consideration of another's time did not exist in his conceited cave. It seems he is now forced to endure all those moments he stole. He lies there for many reasons. Reasons he now defines as sins. Overwhelmed with actions that seemed normal at the time, he now realizes were mistakes that will affect his final score.

Mom feeds him, and I sit in death, breathe death, as it creeps into the foundation of our home.

I'm not surprised he is going to die here. This house is his rock. It warmed and calmed him. I never knew Dad to be strong. In fact, now he is the strongest I have ever seen him, and he can't even get out of the bed. Being home hides his frailness somewhat. The foundation of this house is much sturdier than the foundation of his soul. What he needs to comprehend is the infrastructure of his new home.

Mom is in bed, and I lie next to him, again.

"Molls, are you going to stay here with me?"

"Yeah, Dad. We are going to go to sleep now. I'm right here."

"Okay Skeets, but maybe we should say a prayer first."

"All right Dad, go ahead."

He doesn't respond. I wait a few more seconds, "Dad, I thought you were going to pray?"

Day 23

The morning is bitter cold, as I curl up in the chair, up from the floor after another sleepless night.

"Molly, where's Mom?"

"Dad, she is sleeping, it's only seven."

"It's morning, she needs to get up."

"No, you need to get some sleep. You were up all night. Now go nite-nites."

"Dammit Molly, we need to get up, and I need to take a shower. Go get Ma."

"Dad, you can't take a shower. You are not getting out of the bed. The only way you are getting out of that bed is to let go and accept."

He yells back, "Accept what?"

After a pause I finally breathe the word, "Death, Dad. Accept death."

"When we gonna' have breakfast? Get your mom up so she can make something to eat."

"You just don't want to talk about it do you?"

"Molly, I'm hungry and I want to eat."

"Fine! But don't ask me again to get out of the bed."

I storm to the fridge, lean in, and try to catch my breath. My heart is racing.

"I'm up. I'm up!" Mom says, as she rushes down the hallway.

"Richard, you are a piece of work. Now, what do you want for breakfast?"

"Hi Ma, bacon and eggs sound good."

Mom, already rattled, begins to fritter in the kitchen. I slither downstairs.

After a nice break, my eyes check on him, as my body falls into the chair, and I cuddle up with the remote. I search through the guide and finally choose my channel. In big purple numbers 4-7 appear on the screen. I am filled with fury as I look at The Scene, and then back at the screen—47.

I soon doze off, and sleep in and out, for about two hours.

The phone rings, and I hear Mom say, "Okay, I will open the garage door."

I stretch and rise, "What's going on?"

"Mickey and Lily are here."

I curl up tighter into the blanket and relax.

"We have food, we just came from the store," Mickey's voice fills the house.

I jump up quickly, craving something new.

Mickey hugs me, and says, "Hi kiddo."

He lets go quickly when he notices what is in the living room.

He moves forward, "Hi Dick. You're home."

"Yeah, I'm home, Micks, and it's wonderful."

He approaches The Scene as if it wasn't there, and his hands glide over the rails.

"Boy Dick, you're really crunched up," he says.

"Yeah, I wish there was a way we could get him more in the middle of the bed," I say.

Mickey and Lily help us roll him, but it doesn't help much. Mickey says, "I could lift him up and put him back down."

Mickey cradles Dad's bones and skin. He moans, as he lifts the saggy dead weight.

"Okay Mick, put him down," Lily hollers.

Mickey carefully lets Dad sink into the bed. Trying to catch his breath, he grabs the middle of his back and stretches the kink he just incurred.

*

After a quick moment downstairs, I run up to find a new game and three eager competitors at the table.

For a moment, I forget what is truly at hand, and enjoy the mirage. The game continues, and as we play, we live in the moment of the game. However, this moment is short.

"Molly, I need a pillow under my crack."

"Okay Dad, we will be right there. Let me finish my turn."

We play out the hand because no one sees the importance of a dying man's crack.

"Please Molly, roll me so my hinder doesn't hurt so much."

"All right, Dad. Come on guys, we need to help him."

Lily gets up and shuffles to The Scene, "Okay Dick, what do you want us to do?"

"My hinder is killing me. I need you to slide a pillow under there, and maybe ease the pressure a little bit."

"Come on guys. Let's do this," Lily commands.

Mom growls, "Oh Dick, we just got you situated."

"Tweets, my crack is in so much pain, it's unbearable for me to lie here. Please help me."

"Oh Richard, you have so many issues. You need so much attention."

"All right Mom, come on, put the pillow under him," I groan, as Mickey and I turn him over.

Mom shoves the pillow in there good, and he sighs, "Oh yeah, that's good. Now go back to your game and I'll leave you alone."

We are lost in the enjoyment of the game, but soon interrupted by the sound of the front door opening.

Claire walks in and barely utters, "Hi."

Her voice has always been too soft, not in a cute way, but in a more pathetic, solemn tone. She unties her baby blue trench coat. The sight sends me back to another moment, one I have never recalled, until now.

I was young, maybe second grade, and Dad took me out of school in the middle of the day. He was in a hurry. He picked me up and carried me as he ran down the long olive green hallway from my classroom, out the doors, and into the car. We drove over to a house with lots of trees. We got out and walked in the back door into the kitchen. Jed, Claire's husband, was standing there with a black bag on the floor in front of him.

He said to Dad, "I can't do it, she's back there."

Dad walked to the back. Jed grabbed the bag and walked me to the car, telling me to get in the back seat. Dad walked out with Claire, who was in a powder blue robe. Dad told Jed to put me in front. Jed opened my door and I ran up with Dad. Claire got in the back and Jed shut the door. We drove forever, without any conversation. We pulled into a long driveway up to a big white house; two guys in white came out to help Claire out of the car. I thought to myself, 'why is she in that robe?' I couldn't understand why she wasn't in regular clothes.

When Kate told the story about Dad taking Curtis out of school to take Buck to rehab, I knew it was too familiar. Different characters, but the stories are the same. Twice when given the shot, he failed proper execution. Today's drab fairways are not the first. I've been at his side before, but the more I recall, the more I understand his game. With a bit of scrambling, and a lot of luck, he was not punished for his poor decisions. In his death, the holes are different. Luck does not exist with truth.

Claire approaches the bed, and whimpers, "Hi Dad. It's Claire, how you feelin'?"

"Claire, is that you?"

"Yeah Dad."

"Oh Claire, I'm in constant pain."

"Oh Dad, I'm so sorry. I'm not sure why this is happening? You definitely don't deserve this."

Most would think she was the one about to lose her life.

The door opens, and Bridgett enters and says, "Hey, what's going on?"

Her husband Blake follows her in, carrying the baby. Claire grabs Hunter from Blake, "Let's go see Grandpa."

Bridgett walks up to the table, "What are you doing?"

Mom replies, "Oh, it's a real fun game. You wanna' play?"

"Yeah, sure, let me get a beer and say hi to Gramps."

Bridgett opens her beer as she approaches The Scene, "Hi Gramps, how you doin' today?"

"Hi Bridges, my hinder is killing me. My crack is sore."

"Yeah, all the lying around will do that. Looks like you are propped up well with all those pillows, though."

"Yeah, they take good care of me here."

"It's good you are home."

"You can say that again, Bridges."

Minutes go by as if it was a normal day.

We enjoy today, and he absorbs our sounds. He reacts to everyone coming through the door; it goes both ways. He is saying goodbye.

"We've got to go Mickey. We've been here all day," Lily gets up and approaches Dad.

"Okay Dick, we have to go. You take care, okay? We will be back next week," she leans in and kisses him.

Will this be the last time they see him, or will they circle this bed many more times?

Mickey hugs me tightly, "Hang in there, kiddo."

Lily takes his place and whispers, "You call us, okay?"

The door opens and Mickey yells out, "Bye Dick. We'll see you soon."

"Okay Mick, goodbye."

Lily finishes a hug with Mom, and she yells as she steps out the door, "Bye Dick. We love you."

*

Everyone is finally gone. I sink into my usual spot; the

television breaks the silence of the room. I stare at Dad.

In his final days we are twined together too tightly – so distant, yet too close for comfort.

Mom is in the kitchen. She may have a bit of a compulsive disorder when it comes to the kitchen sink. She wipes it down more in an hour than she wipes her own ass in a week. The poor sink has washcloth burns.

I, on the other hand, sit right in the middle of The Scene. I spend my time watching him, trying to understand his thoughts. I don't dare move my lips to ease any pain. I am terrified of words.

He lies there, and suffers. He sulks in the sorrows of his days, and worries about the ones to come.

In this mediocre moment, silence breathes. We are engrossed in a routine that leaves us speechless. This ridiculous behavior is exhausting. To believe death can be simple is not allowed. His progression I will live and his life I will know.

"Here you go, Molls," Mom says, as she hands me a bowl of stew.

"What about Dad?"

"I got his coming right now."

It takes me a while to eat, as I watch the live dinner theatre.

Dad hollers out, "What is that?"

"It's a carrot, Dick," Mom shouts back.

"Cut it in half. I can't eat that whole thing."

I yell at her, "Mom, you have to be careful. Cut it all up into little pieces."

She breaks the food up and says, "It's just like having a baby."

"Come on, Tweets. I'm hungry."

"Okay, Dick. These are all big chunks. Now, you can wait while I cut them."

He finally gets his bite, and minutes go by while he chews it down.

"How is it?" Mom asks.

His mouth is moving rapidly as though he has the side of a cow inside it, but all he holds is a mere potato piece.

"My God, Dick, you are slow."

"Tweets, I'm old and I'm sick."

"How is it, Richard?"

"It's good, but it's cold."

"You want me to warm it up, Dick."

"That would be nice, Tweets."

Mom walks back into the kitchen. She says under her breath, "Pampered like a baby too."

At the very beginning we are sheltered in a womb, innocent. Protection and nourishment strengthen our form, until we are born into an existence of turmoil and defeat. Our core is tested throughout life, while the body is corrupted with disorder. Before death, guilt invades. The shell is tainted, but the life inside breathes a chance for rebirth of purity.

I stare at him.

Mom and I should be more compassionate with him. We're just over it. A selfish, cheap asshole, that's all I remember of him growing up. I am actually thinking of a way to kill him. Maybe I could put something in his food. He is going to die anyway. So what's the point of him lying there? He could continue his selfish ways and live another couple months, for what? So he can die?

I don't understand why he won't talk to me. What is he thinking? It's not about him or what he did, but it's what he seeks that's important.

Mom finally sits down to relax.

"How gross!" Mom hollers out.

"What?" I say.

"Those two girls just kissed."

"Oh, Mom, get over it already."

"But it's the Academy Awards," she explains.

The door opens and Gabe walks in, "Hello! How is Mr. Richard tonight?"

He approaches The Scene. He rests his hand gently on Dad's shoulder and whispers, "Hi Dick. How are you feeling tonight?"

Dad's eyes open wide, his head turns, and he recognizes the face.

"Oh. Hi Gabe, I am stuffed from a wonderful dinner my beautiful wife made, and now we are watching the Academy Awards."

"Sounds like you are having a good night."

Day 24

The doorbell wakes me up. My eyes open and I reconstruct myself for the start of another day of madness. I stretch vigorously before walking to The Scene.

Amy is standing over Dad.

"Morning," she says, smiling.

I put on the bright teal gloves and tend to the hole in the side of my dad's chest. I do this as though I've done it for years. Mom walks out from the laundry room with clean sheets, and says, "We need to change those sheets because they are full of blood from his sores."

I ask her, "What did Gabe say about the night?"

"He said they talked about God."

I yell back, "They did?"

Mom asks Dad, "Dick, what did you and Gabe talk about last night?"

"We talked about a lot of things, Tweets."

"Gabe told me you talked about God. What did you talk about, Dick?"

He snipes back, "I can't remember all the things he said. Now, I'm hungry. When we gonna' eat?"

I walk into the kitchen to wash my hands and Mom says, "Man, he just won't let go. You can't even get him to talk."

"Yeah, he has major issues. Maybe we should call Pastor out to talk to him. I think he could lie there for a while."

"Oh Molly, don't say that. I need him to let go."

"He's too scared."

"He's always been like that."

I nod my head, "I know. I know."

I walk back to the bed, as Amy says, "We can change the sheets now."

Mom stands to the side of me and together we pull him toward us.

"God dammit, that hurts. You guys need to be gentle with me."

"We are trying, Dad. Give us a break, already. For someone who talked about God last night, you sure are mean today."

"Gabe talked about God, I just listened."

I'm getting upset. My voice cracks, "Well, did you hear anything important?"

"I don't know Molls. Now, will you put me back down?"

Amy's voice rises, "Hold on, I'm trying to take care of a couple irritations."

"So, what did Gabe say, Dick?" Mom says.

"God dammit, Tweets, don't be a such a donkey nuts. Can't you see I got issues?"

"You sure do. You've got major issues."

"All done. You can put him down," Amy says.

Mom and I roll him back as softly as we can.

"Okay, you're all set now Dad."

"Does this mean we are going to eat now?"

Mom screams, "My God, Dick, you are so demanding."

"I'm hungry, Tweets. I haven't had anything to eat since last night."

"Okay Richard, I'll get your breakfast right now."

"Thanks Tweets, and some pop."

I feed him.

He yearns for inner peace and until he has it, he will lie in the bed, distressed. His misery will intensify my misery, Mom's misery, and together we will all be miserable.

Back in the kitchen, I say to Mom, "Okay, I'm going to call Pastor and ask him to come out. Dad's issues are more complicated than we can handle. Then again, we can't handle shit."

I grab the phone and go into the laundry room. I dial the number confidently, but I have no idea what I will say. Pastor answers the phone, "Hi Pastor, it's Molly."

"Hi Molly, how is your dad?"

"Well, I think he has some spiritual issues, and he won't talk about it. I thought maybe you could come out and talk to him."

"I can come out this afternoon, around three."

"That would be great. Thank you so much."

I guess this proves, when we have nowhere else to turn, we turn to God. I have not met God. I do not know what he looks like. I've seen pictures in books – the white beard and the white robe. But, I have not seen him in person. I try not to talk to him either, because he never talks back. My mother and father created me. I know them, they talk to me, and they are here on Earth, but God is not. I must be out of options. Maybe Pastor can ease his anger and help him understand what death means.

When I return to the living room Mom is in her chair with her mouth wide open, snoring loudly.

I grab a blanket and cling to the mattress on the floor. I am silent, aware of everything around me. Dad's eyes are open, but I'm not sure if he is conscious of his surroundings.

*

Mom is now on the phone, and I try to find something for entertainment on the television.

Dad calls out, "Hey Molls, the Hallmark channel always has on good shows."

"Mom, what channel is Hallmark?"

"Two-sixteen, Molls. I'm on the phone with Aunt Susan."

I check the guide to see what is on the requested channel, and of course, it's a movie that takes place in the year 1947.

"Okay Dad, this looks good for now. I'm going to go downstairs and take a shower."

My feet hit the floor solidly and another leap gets me to the bottom of the stairs. I sprint to the bathroom and prepare my pipe with a bit of grass. I inhale deeply and step into the shower. I exhale, letting the hard streams of water hit my face.

I find myself on the couch downstairs, interested in the coffee table. It is a big wooden square with slide out drawers and a glass top that displays ribbons, medals, pictures, and newspaper clippings of my junior golf career. I pull out the top drawer to study the shrine.

Soon all the drawers are emptied, and my high school golf paraphernalia is everywhere around me. I'm reading the fifth of many articles written about me, and I'm surprised my parents are not mentioned. The stories are all about my game, my shots, and even my practice routines. All my quotes are the same—technical, but in no way emotional. Normally, when it comes to sports, a father is mentioned.

"Molly, Molly, Pastor is here!"

Mom's scream alarms me; I jump to my feet and sprint up the stairs.

I approach the living room, unsure of what to expect.

Pastor says, "Hi Molly."

"Hello."

Mom, without hesitation, says, "Pastor, we think Dick is having spiritual issues."

Pastor walks toward The Scene and asks, "What are your concerns, Dick?"

Dad's voice crinkles, "How can a guy like me ask the Lord to go to Heaven?"

Pastor replies, "Do you believe in Jesus Christ?"

"Yes."

"Have you asked him for forgiveness?"

"Yes."

"Well, then you have nothing to worry about."

"But what if my sins were bad?"

Pastor smiles and shakes his head, "Dick, everybody sins, you are not the only one. Nobody would even be in Heaven because we all sin, but the ones who accept Christ and seek his forgiveness will have eternal life. Let me tell you a story about Jesus, a cross, a thief, and what you desire most—forgiveness."

He begins the saga and I'm intrigued by it. It represents my father completely.

"Jesus hung on a cross between two thieves, both hurling abuse, but soon one became humble with regret. He admitted to rebuking his fellow mankind and conceded that his suffering was just."

I look at Dad.

He is the thief, stuck in the bed, waiting to die. He knows he did wrong but he fights and pleads for salvation.

Pastor says, "And the thief says to Jesus, 'Remember me when you come into your Kingdom!'"

He then grabs Dad's hand and asks, "Dick, do you know what Jesus said back to the thief?"

"No," Dad whispers.

"Well, Jesus said to him, 'Truly, I say to you, today you shall be with me in paradise.'"

Silence calms the room.

Pastor soon continues, "Dick, you had a fantastic life, surrounded with love from your family. You are surrounded by love now, and soon you are going to a place where there is even more love. It's so much better we can't even imagine it. Its beauty is beyond anything we can comprehend. The vividness and the colors are more than our eyes can see. Can you imagine it, Dick?"

Dad thinks for a moment and says, "Well, you are right about one thing: I do have a wonderful family. But to answer your question, No, I can't imagine Heaven, but I can imagine Hell."

Mom and I smirk. She asks, "Do you think you feel this way because of what you did for a living?"

Dad responds, "Yeah."

Mom says, "Because you owned a bar?"

Come on Mom, really?

He gives the familiar one word answer, "Yeah."

Pastor interjects, "A sin is a sin whatever it is, and everyone sins. Nobody is special. We are all sinners. It's what we do about it, and how we accept it."

Dad responds, "Are you sure about a guy like me?"

Mom and I sigh, defeated.

Pastor says, "Let's say a prayer."

We grab hands around the bed.

Pastor begins, "Dear Lord—"

All I can think about is the war on my father's soul. I just saw it with my own two eyes. The Pastor, a representative of God, and Dad's corrupted being, debating words of salvation. I am very worried for my father; he needs to understand Pastor's words.

Pastor continues, "Richard is opening his soul to you, Lord. Please grant him forgiveness, and allow peace to take over this house and family. Reinforce in Richard the beauty of your home that we call Heaven. We pray for his salvation, for your arms to embrace him, so he may live with you, Lord, in eternal peace. Amen."

Dad says to Pastor, "Can I ask you one more question?"

"Sure."

"What holiday is more important, Christmas or Easter?"

"Easter is much more significant. The resurrection of Christ is the holiest day of all."

Dad, like a child, says, "It is?"

Pastor announces, "Yes, of course."

*

He is calm. Mom is in the kitchen cooking dinner. The news is on. Big white numbers drown the screen. I yell at Mom, "Look."

The five-day forecast comes up, and I blurt, "Oh, keep in mind, it's supposed to be forty-seven degrees Thursday, Friday, and Saturday too."

An animated movie about sled dogs comes on. I know this movie is old because I remember we watched it together, probably about twenty years ago.

It was a night much like tonight, cold outside, Mom in the kitchen and Dad in his brown chair, wearing his brown corduroys, brown turtleneck, and brown boots.

"When's dinner gonna' be ready?" he shouts.

"It's coming Dick," Mom hollers. "Here Molls, come and get Dad's dinner."

I let the cartoon voices carry me off, as I put the fork into his mouth, wait, put the fork in his mouth, wait, put the fork in his mouth, and wait. When this becomes unbearable, I turn my eyes to the television and take in the bright colors. A character says, "Forty-seven goose eggs would be fantastic."

"Molls, Molly, come on Molls," Dad's voice destroys my stillness as I give him another forkful.

"How is it, Dad?"

"It's good, but it's cold."

"It's cold?"

"Well, it's not hot."

"You want me to warm it up?"

"Yeah."

As I approach the kitchen, Mom asks, "Now what?"

"He says it's cold."

"He is unbelievable."

He screeches, "Hey Molls."

"Yeah, Dad."

"Put more gravy in there, Skeeters."

Mom groans, "God, he is so needy, I wish he would just let go."

I respond, "I think it's going to be a while."

"Oh Molly, don't say that."

"He has too many issues, and he just doesn't want to face them."

Day 27

The house has been still. There hasn't been much movement within the rails for the past couple of days. This is the quietest Dad has been so far. Perhaps he is absorbing Pastor's words.

His shirt is stained badly from the tumor drainage, so I carefully remove it from his arm. Amy says, "Spray a lot of it," as she hands me the bottle of cancer cleaner.

The mass soaks in white foamy bubbles. The shape has changed: it is bigger, wider on all sides, it now covers his nipple. The skin above is hard and solid, but the tissue within is decaying, and bigger pieces of the sponge-like substance stick to the gauze.

"That's crazy," I say, as I wiggle the gauze over the wastebasket, watching a grape-sized piece of his chest dangle from the bandage.

Mom says, "Molly, that's disgusting."

I turn back to his chest. The lining of the deformity is light beige, dried up, and bare. It crumbles. The inner core is bright—red muscle pumping little green trenches of poison.

It looks like a desert city with the brown of the mountains on the outside, and the flesh-eating, life-sucking day-by-day world on the inside.

I doubled the materials that I thought would prevent leakage, and used almost three times as much tape, trying to seal his wicked wound.

*

It feels nice to be dressed and ready to go into the world.

It still exists, even though I haven't been a part of it for days.

I make my way up and into the kitchen. My eyes flash to a blue object on the counter and I say, "Why is that there?"

Mom says, "What?"

I reply, "The hair dryer."

Mom says, "I found it in the garbage."

I laugh as I ask, "And why do you think it was in there?"

She replies, "You can still use it."

I shake my head and explain, "Mom, it was smoldering in my hand. Flames were coming out of it. It's broken, done. Now, I'm throwing it out."

I grab it and set it in the trash can.

Mom is putting on her jacket, as Dad says, "Tweets, you shouldn't be going out. You should stay here with me."

"Richard, we have to get out of this house. Now, you better be good."

He yells back, "God dammit Tweets, you are spending money when you could just stay here with me."

The doorbell rings, and I hurry to let Dee in.

Mom points her finger almost to his nose and says, "Dick, I mean it. Don't you be naughty."

He screams, "You always were a donkey nuts, Tweets!"

*

We pull into the driveway after being out all day. Mom says, "Shoot, we can't get in the garage."

The lights shine on the two cars in front of us, and the glow of the numbers off the white metal stings my eyes.

"Oh my God, look!" I say.

Mom replies, "What?"

I explain, "The license plates on both of them have a forty-seven. Look, that's just stupid."

Mom sees what I see. Her mouth drops, "That is weird."

A knock on the window startles us. I open the car door. Leslie says, "Hey, I'm leaving. I have to get to class, but I will be back tomorrow."

I shut the door, and Mom backs the car up as she says, "You know, Leslie was born in 1947 too."

"Of course she was."

I run straight downstairs from the car. I need to chill before I approach The Scene. I look in the mirror, puff, and inhale deeply. Mom's voice is loud, but her words are muddled. Then an angry yell echoes through the foundation.

"Jesus Christ, now what?" I scream, sprinting out of the bathroom and back up the stairs.

"What the hell is going on up here?" I say, moving

quickly to The Scene.

Mom replies, "He doesn't understand why we need home care."

"Tweets, I just don't see the point of paying money to have someone here when you can take care of me," Dad yells.

My eyes meet his and I say, "Okay, Dad here's the deal. We need the home care because we can't do it alone. You wanted to come home, and you are home. You can either drop the home care issue, or you can go back to the nursing home."

"Okay Molls. I'm just voicing my opinion. You guys don't give me a chance to say anything."

I laugh, "Are you kidding? You never say anything to begin with. You won't even talk about it. What do you suggest we do, Dad?"

"I agree with you, Skeets."

"Good, now why won't you talk to us? We are here, Mom and me, now let's have a conversation."

"I said what I said when Pastor was here. I'm just not ready yet."

"That's fine, but we need help. You are home, and we are in charge. This is how it is going to be. So please, I don't want to hear about the home care again."

He has no response, but I can tell he has something to say.

"Would you like to talk to either of us privately?"

He whimpers, "I already did. I told your mom I loved her, and I had a great family. I told you when the Pastor was here how blessed I was."

I grab his hand, there are tears running off his puffy

cheeks.

"Dad, it's okay."

Mom grabs his other hand.

"Oh Richard, everything is going to be fine, you have to have faith."

He whines, "I do. I told you when the Pastor was here."

I say, "We just want you to be able to tell us anything, if you want to. We just want you to talk to us, tell us what you are thinking."

He pauses for a long moment. Mom and I look at each other.

"I think I want a cookie."

I yell, "Seriously, that's it! That's what you have to say? Wow!"

I throw my hands in the air and walk toward the kitchen, "What the hell is wrong with you?"

Mom follows behind me and mutters, "I don't know how much longer I can take this."

*

After being quiet for hours, he breaks the silence.

"Get me the fuck out of here," he wails.

Mom says, "What did you just say, Richard?"

"You heard me. Get me the fuck out of here, and put me to bed."

He is twitching.

"I need to get outta' this fucking bed. Come on, let's go mother fucker, get me outta' here."

His body is turned to the left bedrail. Both hands clench the steel as he pulls himself up. Hatred drives him.

Mom whimpers, "Why are you acting like this? Why are you being so mean?"

He groans, "Asshole. You always were a smart ass. Get me out of this fuckin' bed, now!"

Gabe walks through the door, "Hello?"

He quickly comes to assist.

Dad is calming down. He is on his back again and his hands are resting in his lap. He whispers, "I see light."

His right hand extends up. Gabe says, "That's good."

Mom asks, "What do you see, Dick?"

His hand is still high while his fingers grab onto the air. He answers, "It's a normal looking guy."

His index finger points, "Look Tweedles, it's God, I see God."

"How do you know it's God? What does he look like?"

His voice is weak, his words are soft, "He looks like the neighbor, he is so normal, like me."

I look at Gabe; his smile and nod tell me this could be the start of something good.

Dad hollers, "I think I'm going to get to go to Heaven."

The radiance upon his face dims, as he ponders aloud, "But I can't go yet, because I need to see the Big Guy first, and I don't know what to say."

Mom says, "It's okay, Richard. You can go."

Gabe says, "This is good, but he could struggle for a few more weeks."

"Weeks?" I retort.

"The way he is fighting, I wouldn't be surprised."

Dad shouts, "Get me the fuck out of here. If you don't put me to bed, I'm gonna' rip your fuckin' head off!"

Mom looks confused, "I don't understand, how did he change like that?"

Gabe says, "You may want to call the nurse. He is very agitated."

Over the phone the hospice nurse, Courtney, gives me directions for giving him the drops.

"Okay Dad, this should make you feel better. Open your mouth."

As instructed, I drop it in his gums and then rub his cheek.

Mom is at the table reading the hospice book.

I ask Gabe, "What is happening?"

Gabe replies, "He sees Heaven and he feels the hate of Hell. He admitted he couldn't face God, yet. He is struggling spiritually."

Dad starts to twitch and yell, "Help me. Please help me."

Mom runs over and says, "Richard, go toward the light. Do you see the light?"

His hand reaches out high and he whispers, "Yeah."

He calms down, staring at the ceiling, but every so often jerks with a cry for help. I take his hand through the cold steel rail. Gabe says, "Go toward God, Richard. He is waiting for you."

Whatever is going on, it is real. I can feel its presence.

We've been sitting here for hours. Each of us conveying comfort, hoping soon he will take our advice and seek the light.

He cries out, "Help me. Help me go to sleep."

"It's okay, Dad. You can go to sleep, just relax."

His eyes are really big as they look up toward the ceiling, and with delight he whispers, "I see him, I see him. God almighty is over there."

Mom, drunk with fatigue, utters back to him, "Richard, you can go now. It's time to go to sleep."

I give him the next dose of drops and say, "Okay Dad, this is going to help you sleep."

"How am I going to sleep when I'm not in the bed?" he screams.

"You are in the bed."

"God dammit, don't be a fucking tease. I'm not in my bed. Take me to bed."

Mom says, "What a one-eighty he does. He sees the light one minute and the next minute he is awful."

Gabe explains, "He is angry because he sees Heaven, but he can't get to it. He realizes he is back on Earth, after he has seen where he could be."

I enter the kitchen and the green neon digits glare at me, I say, "Oh my God, it's almost three in the morning."

Mom yells, "No, really?"

"Two-forty seven, to be exact."

Conditions are changing. The holes are getting longer. The clouds are rolling in. We have been in the thick, wet rough most of the round, definitely not in the fairway. Now there is trouble beyond the rough – sand, bushes, and trees. The course is too narrow for his mistakes. He is all over the place, leaving himself with almost impossible shots.

Golf is an individual sport with many rules. Some play by the book, counting every single stroke, and penalize themselves even when alone. Others are aware of the rules, but break them anyway. In the end, we are left lying in a bed in the living room, dying; trying to recognize God in ourselves, to sign an honest scorecard.

Day 28

I explain the night we had to Heather, and tell her that I gave him the drops for the first time. She says, "It's time to stop his pills. He is now in the dying process, so he will only use the drops. As soon as he shows signs of restlessness, or gets upset in any way, give him one of each drop, immediately."

Mom is combing his hair. He says to her, "I have to go, I have a tee time."

Mom asks, "You do, with who?"

He returns, "Jimmy M."

Mom's mouth drops, but she recovers quickly, "Jimmy M? You have a tee time with Jimmy M?"

He doesn't respond, but makes another request, "Are you going to get me something to eat? I'm hungry Tweets."

Jimmy M was the first of Dad's good friends to die. He too died of a heart attack while on the golf course. I remember Kate saying Jimmy was even worse than Dad with the women. They went to Arizona all the time together, and I'm sure they had their fun.

After a few bites of oatmeal Mom tries once more, "Dick, did you see Jimmy M?"

Frustrated, he complains, "You and your fucking questions. I waited in the car for seven hours for you to come home."

Mom and I can't help but chuckle. Our squirmy giggles displease him more. He shouts, "Don't be so fucking smart. I'll be glad when I'm dead and gone."

I say to him, "Well, where you are going is a lot better than here. You can go, you should. You will be much happier."

He ignores my comment, and refuses his next spoonful. Mom says, "Come on Dick, take it."

He whines, "I don't want it. I want something else."

Mom moans back, "What do you want, Dick?"

"A cheeseburger."

"You want a cheeseburger for breakfast?"

"Oh, don't be such a donkey nuts, Tweets. You asked me what I want, and I want a cheeseburger."

"I don't have a cheeseburger, Dick. You are going to have to wait. What about an orange?"

"Yeah, and ice cream."

Once he is finished eating, he asks, "Molls, can you move the TV over?"

"What? What do you mean?"

"Move it in front of me."

"It is in front of you, can't you see it?"

"Yeah Skeets, but it needs to be adjusted better."

"Well, I can move you maybe, but I can't change the TV."

I tilt the head of the bed up, move his pillows, and adjust his body. I am out of breath, "There, how is that, Dad?"

"I can't see the television screen, Molly. You need to angle the TV better."

I point to the television, it is about ten feet directly in front of him.

"Dad, it is right here. Do you see it?"

He doesn't respond.

"Dad, Dad, over here. Can you see the TV, Dad?"

He seems oblivious.

"Okay Dad, I give up. I need to go to the bathroom, I will be right back."

I try to chill, but can't concentrate. I hear his voice all the way in this corner, below the floorboards.

"Ma, Ma, Ma," penetrates the walls.

Quick to his need, I run up the stairs and yell, "What is going on up here?"

He screams, "Where is your mom. I ask her for something and don't get it for thirty minutes."

I come back, "First of all, you can wait because you did at the nursing home, all the time. And second of all, you will wait because Mom is busy right now."

He cries back, "You're my daughter. You are supposed to be nice to me."

"I'm here taking care of you, aren't I?"

"Take my coat off God dammit, but tell your mom we are going home soon."

Babe opens the door and says, "Here is Wrigley. Sorry, we are running late, see you later."

Wrigley runs to me, and jumps on my lap.

Thank God Wrigley is here to lighten things up.

*

I get in the car with Wrigley, and turn the key. The neon green time reads 1:47. I turn to the pup and say, "Oh Wriggers, what a crock of shit."

He looks at me with excitement, and I realize he is right. I should be happy to go for this drive. It is the first time I have driven a car in nearly a month. Almost thirty days have gone by, and I still have no understanding of the situation.

I see the gas station, "Sweet, Wriggers, let's get some cash, in case Uncle Mick decides to bring me more weed."

Wriggers looks up at me. His eyes say, *sounds good to me.*

I pull in and go inside to the ATM machine. There is a man with a tape measure trying to measure a set of drink coolers. My transaction is complete, but the man is having difficulty with his task. I approach him and ask, "Can I help you?"

He replies, "Oh, yes, thank you. Just hold this here."

He hands me the tape measure and then pulls the tape away from me. He stretches his head toward me while he looks down at the end of the tape in my hand, and reads, "Forty-seven inches. Thank you very much."

"No problem, anytime."

I turn around, walk out to the car, open the door, and get in. My head falls to the steering wheel as I say, "Last time I do anyone a favor. How is that even possible?"

Wrigley's head tilts back and forth while I ramble on, "I mean forty-seven inches. It has to be some sort of sign, Wriggers."

Wrigley steps up on my lap, and for the first time, I feel like someone is listening.

*

I hear loud voices as I walk through the door. I yell out, "I have your cheeseburger."

Mom says, "He is being nasty right now."

He screams, "You sure like to get your fucking cookies off. I would hit you, but they would haul me off to jail."

"What the hell is he talking about?" I ask.

He shouts, "I want her to get me out of this fucking bed. She thinks it's funny I can't get out."

I respond, "She doesn't think it's funny. Dad, she can't help you get out. You are never getting out of this bed, ever, at least not your body. Your soul, I'm not sure, because it seems destroyed by something. If I were you, I would free your demons now."

He doesn't respond, so I shove the cheeseburger into his mouth. The big bite is followed by many seconds to devour it. He looks like a baby with an old man's face. His infant cry contradicts his wrinkled skin as he groans, "Where is the frosty?"

"It's here Dad. God, finish chewing, already!

He is so much different than yesterday. For the first time, he is not making any sense.

"Skeets, did you take the pipe out of the well?"

"Yeah Dad. It's all good."

"Don't be a smart ass, and help me get out of this bed."

I run downstairs, but within minutes I can hear his screams, "Ma, Ma, Ma!"

I run back up to heed his call, "What Dad? What is it?"

He screams, "Get your mom, so I can get out of this fucking bed. Please Molly, help me, don't be such a donkey nuts."

If he can get out of the bed he thinks he can get out of the situation. He is stranded; can't hide from anything. It is his only hope of freedom from what faces him.

Mom has disappeared. It's a bit warmer today; she must have retreated to the yard. I eat my food and watch from a distance, but not *too* far. He hollers out, "Molly, how is Dirk Riffling doing?"

I reply, "Not very well, I hear."

Dad's friend Dirk is also very ill; doctors told him he was terminal years ago.

They have been friends since they were kids. He came into The Avenue all the time. He was the fat alcoholic who sat at the end of the bar. You could estimate his tab by his weight. How many free drinks make up a pound? Most say, Riffling is a bit of a con. He was an insurance salesman, and fit the part.

I never got into too much trouble with Dad. However, one time I recall Dad screaming at me when it wasn't even my fault. The fridge in the garage was always filled with beer. Most of Dad's golfing buddies would help stock it, and then dwindle it back as they played. Riffling was the guy who filled it the least, but opened it the most. It was a Saturday, and we were out for the day. Dad normally left the side door unlocked so his pals could have access to a cold treat at all times. Accidentally, the door was locked, and Riffling felt he had no choice but to break it down to fulfill his desire. Dad did not know that right away. He thought I was the one who broke the door. He was mad at me for a few days, until another friend revealed that it was Dirk. But he never confessed. To this day, I bet he would deny it. Riffling lingers in death as well.

Lynn and Mom walk in the house. Mom says, "Come on Molly, we are going to play Hand and Foot."

Dad yells out, "Molly, I want to go to bed."

Mom yells back, "You are in bed, Richard."

He moans, "Oh, not you and your bullshit. I'm not talking to you."

Zack walks in, and says, "Oh God, the girls and their cards."

Zack was always one of my favorite of Dad's friends. This is probably because he is one of the youngest of the group. Today he is sixty. He has always been stocky, but his stomach is definitely bigger than I remember. His hair is still brown, but I can't tell how much of it exists, since he always wears a ball cap.

He walks over to Dad and asks, "Weasel, how the hell are you sitting here with no golf on, listening to these women?"

Dad replies, "They're a bunch of assholes."

Mom shouts, "Richard, that's enough."

He hollers back, "I asked you to put me to bed. Now, do you think you could please help me?"

"Dick, I have told you, you are in your bed."

He says angrily, "I love you so much, and you treat me like shit."

I put the drop of medicine against his gum.

He says to Mom, "I'm an old fart. I can't take this abuse."

She replies, "Go nite-nites."

"Oh, I wish I could, Tweedles, I wish I could."

He asks Zack, "Do you have an extra bed at your house?"

"Yeah, we have a couple."

"Well, do you think you could wheel me down to your house, so I can get some sleep?"

"Why don't you just go to sleep here?"

"I would, but those assholes won't take me to bed."

"Yeah, those assholes," Zack concurs.

Lynn yells, "Zack, don't agree with him."

Dad yells out, "Molly's mom is an asshole."

Mom, Lynn, and I move to Dad's side. He hollers out, "Hey Zack, how come I'm getting all the lovin' over here, and you ain't gettin' shit."

Zack chuckles back, "I'm used to it Weasel, it's okay."

Lynn sighs, "Oh, I love you Dick. You are so special."

His voice softens, "I'm gonna' go to sleep now."

Lynn tells him, "Take some deep breaths and relax. Just go off to dreamland for a bit."

*

Mom and I doze off. An hour later the phone rings, and he goes berserk.

He screams, "Get off the fuckin' phone!"

Mom replies, "I'm on the phone with your daughter, Claire."

Her comeback silences him for a second, then, "Ma, Ma."

She ignores his plea.

He screams even louder, "God damn, you fuck around more than a barrel of monkeys. Please help me, Ma. Please."

I ask, "Dad, what do you need?"

"I'm gonna' burn this fuckin' house down if she doesn't get off that fuckin' phone."

He wiggles around frantically and shouts, "Come on Ma! Get the papers above the cab on the passenger side of the truck."

Mom is not paying any attention to him.

"Come on, Molly!"

"What do you want, Dad?"

"Mom needs to get in the truck, sign the papers, and we need to go. Get your mom off the fuckin' phone."

"Dad, Mom is talking to Claire, now just hold on a minute."

Louder he cries, "Come on Ma! For Christ sake, please help me get outta' here. Get off the phone. I don't want her talking to her. She can talk to Babe, but not her. Molly, get her off the phone, now!"

I finally say to Mom, "You need to get off the phone because I need to call hospice."

A little softer, Dad asks, "Molly, will you pile me up in the back of the truck?"

Mom says, "Claire is going to bring her Pastor out tomorrow."

I call hospice, and Courtney tells me to give him a bit more of the agitation drops. He has been needy and mean all day, and tonight I have the pleasure of watch duty.

*

I haven't had to get up much, but it is 2:30 a.m. and I'm still wide awake due to his cries, "Ma, Ma, Ma, help me, please, help me. Ma, Ma..."

Day 29

The last twenty-four hours have been the toughest so far. I call hospice to explain that he has been screaming all night, and still this morning. Courtney prescribes a higher dosage of the drops, and this time it actually works.

After a nice break in my sanctuary, I return to find Dirk and Fran Riffling in the living room.

Dirk is wearing sweatpants and a stained tee shirt. I don't think I ever saw him in anything else. His bottoms always had an elastic band with a drawstring, and his shirts were mostly full of rings. His wife is the opposite – petite, neat, and looking much younger than her years.

Dirk's skin is bloodless and blotchy, and he is breathing heavily. He sits in Mom's chair, staring at his pal lying there, collecting himself before approaching the bed. After about twenty minutes, he advances to the dining room chair that I put next to the bed for visitors. He is shaky with his claw cane as he sits down. His fingers tighten on the rail and his knuckles threaten to burst through the case of his meaty hand. With his other hand, he kneads his knee compulsively. His eyes seek the face of his dear friend.

Dad is non-responsive.

Two minutes is all Riffling can bear, he says, "Okay

Fran, it's time to go."

His head turns again toward Dad and drops. Lost in thought, he turns away from the bed trembling. He gets his cane in the right position, and gradually makes his way out the door.

*

It's almost 4:00 p.m., and Dad is awake from his silent state. Claire and her Pastor arrive. Claire says, "I think we should go downstairs and let Pastor Drake talk to Dad."

We follow her down the stairs.

Claire says, "I think if Dad wants to say something, he may feel more comfortable telling Pastor Drake alone."

Mom replies, "Well, what do you think he wants to say?"

"I don't know. That's why I wanted my pastor to come and talk to him."

Waiting down here makes no sense to me. Why does her pastor have to be alone with Dad?

Only seconds later, Pastor Drake's voice calls from the top of the stairs, "Okay, we are finished, you can come back up."

Mom says, "Well, that was fast."

Claire hurries up the stairs. I look at Mom, and roll my eyes, "Seriously?"

I sprint to catch her. I don't want her talking to *anyone* alone.

She says to Pastor Drake, "Did he tell you anything?"

He replies, "No, but everything is fine. When the Lord is ready, He will take him. Your dad says he has asked for forgiveness and salvation. He knows what is going on."

I reply, "You really think so?"

"Yes."

Claire asks, "What else?"

"I don't know. It's in the Lord's hands."

We stand in the kitchen, as Pastor Drake says, "Let's pray together."

He grabs my hand and Claire's, and Mom joins in the middle.

It seems weird because we are not praying with Dad. I'm not listening to the words of the prayer, but here we are again, asking God to take him.

Claire's pastor left, but she sits at the counter, perplexed, "Something doesn't seem right. Poor Dad."

Mom replies, "I think your dad has a lot more issues than we thought."

Mom is correct. This is a new stage in his progression. His eyes were shut almost the entire day. Sleep, however, is not the major task at hand. He is performing self-observation on a plane that doesn't exist to us.

Claire notices the microwave and says, "Hey, Molly, it's 4:47. Does that mean something?"

A bit frustrated, I growl, "I have no idea."

A couple of hours have gone by and I can't believe how tolerable Claire has been. We are watching some crazy game show and, seemingly, enjoying each other's company while doing so. Mom flips the channels and hits one that is playing church music. Dad shouts out, "Leave it there."

The sounds must soothe the spirit and heartache he studies within.

*

Mom and I have enjoyed a few hours alone. Dad has been asleep since Claire left.

I'm tending to the tumor, "Say something to me."

He replies, "I love you."

In shock, I say, "Oh my God, I love you too."

I turn to Mom and smile. "He actually said something

normal."

Mom approaches the bed, "Say something to me."

He says, "I love you."

At the exact same time Mom and I ask, "Can you open your eyes?"

One lid is able to lift. He is weak, and falls right back into the zone that he has been submerged in all day.

Dee arrives and I'm already curled in bed, but I hear him cry, "Help me, Ma, Ma, Ma, Ma, help me. Please put me to bed!"

Dad didn't hit the ball very far, but it was always straight. When he did hit it in the trees it seemed to bounce right back out into the fairway. Even if he hit the ball into the water it would usually skip out, somehow. This in golf lingo is referred to as a 'member's bounce', any favorable bounce of the golf ball improving what initially appeared to be an errant shot. His life was also filled with errors, but no one knew, except the few people in his group who actually witnessed his many member's bounces. In his looming death, all of his mistakes are shown to him. These sins are his prison; he is stuck in the midst of trees. He will keep swinging until he is forced to concede his penalty to get back onto open grass. He sees the green ahead and struggles to move closer to the pin.

Day 30

Organ pipes and opera voices awaken me. It sounds like there is a choir in the kitchen, but it is just Mom near the stove, and the television blaring. I plop in the chair and examine Dad for a moment. His eyes are closed; I do not know what goes on behind them.

Mom walks over and says, "Richard, I need to brush your teeth."

Her toil with what used to be a simple chore is heartbreaking. He is fighting, and she is trying to get him to behave normally. Fed up, she yells, "That's it. What a mess!"

I walk over to him and say, "Dad, will you open your eyes for me?"

Both lids flitter, and then pop open wide. The blue of the sky gazes at me.

Mom comes out with a golf shirt, saying, "I want you to look nice for your kids."

"Shouldn't I take my pills before they get here?" he asks.

"You don't take the pills anymore." Mom replies.

He softly questions, "Why not?"

I reply, "Remember, you have those drops now

instead."

"Oh, okay, I'm going to rest my eyes now."

Sleeping is becoming more and more frequent. He has accepted dying, and is starting to withdraw.

He is out cold another hour before he yells, "Ma! Ma! Get me out of this bed."

Mom replies, "You can't, Richard."

"But I want to sit up."

Mom brings the head of the bed completely up.

"Let's see if the golf is on," she says.

With a cheery voice, he replies, "Yeah."

Now Mom is on the phone, and Dad can hear everything she says.

"Molly thinks he has major issues. I mean, he just won't let go."

I turn to her and say, "Mom, go in the other room and talk."

Of course, she does not take my advice, and continues to converse about the situation.

Dad asks, "Where is the doggie?"

I reply, "What doggie?"

"Wrigley? Where is Wrigley?"

"I will go see if I can get him."

By the time I get back with the dog, Curtis and his kids have arrived, with Claire. I hold up Wrigley in front of Dad, and say, "Here you go."

Dad's hands bury in the dog's fur, as he says, "Hi Wriggs. How are ya', pal?"

We always had dogs. In fact, we always ended up with the neighbors' dogs. Dad's favorite was Duke, a beautiful Irish Setter. Every morning when Dad went to work, Duke would go as well. He would sit behind each green, and wait for Dad to finish mowing down the fairway. Once Dad finished, Duke would run to the next green, and this process continued until all the holes were mowed. Playing in the early morning, I would see Duke with the sun's first rays shining off his red coat, while he sat in the wet dew of the green grass watching his master.

Somehow, Dad is completely normal, responsive, and talking with everyone.

They would never believe me if I relayed the rage he displayed last night. It really pisses me off. We've gone through hell these last few days, but no sign shows through his tame, well-mannered disposition.

Claire says, "Curtis, are you going to say a prayer?"

Curtis puts his plate down, and folds his hands, "Dear God, please, take care of my father. Please, help my father."

He clears his throat, but doesn't continue, due to the tears he can't hold back anymore. All he can bear is, "Amen."

I say to Curtis, "I can't believe he is up and alert. The last couple days he hasn't really been here."

Curtis replies, "Really? He seems fine. Seems to be okay. Way better than when he was at the hospital."

"Well, of course."

I continue to feed Dad and examine the room. Mom is at the counter, alone. Everyone else is at the table, talking.

The clan leaves and Mom and I are alone with Dad again. As we roll him he screams, "Don't do that. God dammit, you're fucking hurting me."

Day 31

It's Monday morning, Oprah is on, and Dad is on a roll. I start removing the tumor dressing.

He yells, "Jesus Christ, Molly! You're hurting me."

We manage to get through the routine, but he is in a lot of pain and pissed as could be, "Get me out this fucking bed, Molly. Come on, God dammit!"

Oprah asks the famous figure, "When did you finally feel at peace with everything?"

The guest answers, "When love overcame fear. Life is lived in distress, until love prevails."

Those words go right through me. I stand in a house full of fear. I turn to him, helpless, and say, "Dad, your love needs to be stronger than your fear. When this happens you will be at peace with yourself, and then you will go to Heaven. I'm sorry Dad, but in order to end your suffering love needs to overcome your fear of death. You need to forgive yourself, Dad, and move on."

He doesn't respond; he never does. He just lies there, miserable, waiting to die.

After a nice break in my sanctuary, I walk back into the

living room.

Mom walks by and says, "I am going downstairs to dry my hair."

I jump in Mom's chair, and say, "Okay."

Dad screams, "Molly, Molly, come here quick, help me."

I jump up, and leap toward The Scene, "What's wrong?"

"I'm stuck, it won't go. I'm trying, but it just won't go. Skeeters, push me to the top of the hill and let go, and maybe I'll go."

I don't respond, I'm not sure how.

He cries out, "Come on, Molly."

I ask him, "Where are we?"

"Oh shit, you're too little, you can't push me. Go get Henry, he can help."

I decide to play along and say, "You're on the hill, you can let go."

He rocks his body back and forth as if he is trying to move the bed. Anger takes over and he yells, "Stupidest thing I've ever seen. Why I can't go, I just don't know."

I had no idea what he meant, but at the same time knew completely what the words stood for.

"Yes it is Dad, I agree."

"Go tell Mom I won't be home for dinner and thanks for helping me."

"Where are you?"

"On top of the seventeenth green."

"The seventeenth green?"

"The mower is stuck, must be a bad battery. I won't make it to the next hole."

Perplexed, I stutter, "Bad battery?"

His hands come together and his fingers begin to squiggle around, then he says to me, "Take these two wires and put them together."

I reach my hands out toward his and pretend to fulfill his request. I say, "Okay Dad, all good. It should work now."

His foot is moving back and forth, "Skeeters, push me forward so my foot can reach the pedal."

I grab the bed remote and move him upright as though he was in the driving position.

He looks at me and pleads, "Molly, please help me. Go get Henry. He can get me out of here."

I look at him with a little grin.

"Molly, this isn't funny! This thing is going to cost $2,000 to get fixed. Bud is going to kill me. Now, please help me."

"Okay Dad, let's go, I think I got it."

His foot is moving again. He screams, "Come on Molly, help me reach the pedal."

His hand starts to wave around in midair. His blue eyes are open wide, mesmerized.

I ask him, "What do you see?"

He breathes, "A light."

"Is it bright?"

"Very bright."

He turns to face me, but his eyes look beyond me,

somewhere off into the distance. They get bigger and bluer as they fixate on whatever it is behind me.

What does he see?

I ask him, but he doesn't respond. He is too intrigued by the vision. I lean toward him and ask him once more, "Dad, what do you see?"

He mumbles something I can't comprehend.

I lean into him really close and whisper, "Dad, what do you see?"

He jumps up and screams in my face, "I see you! God dammit, I see you!"

I bounce back almost to the ground and shout, "Holy fuck."

He yells back, "You scared the shit out of me."

I grab the cold rail tightly, as I catch my breath, "No, you scared the shit out of me."

I pound my feet on the floor to get Mom's attention. Something is going on and I'm not going to face it alone.

He shouts, "Watch it! Watch it! The train is falling off the track."

Mom finally walks in, "Molly, that bathroom is a wreak down there, you've got your marijuana all over the place."

"What? Get over it, already. Didn't you hear me pounding on the floor?"

"No, I was drying my hair."

"He is saying weird things."

Mom walks up to him, "Richard, what are you doing?"

He looks up at her and says, "Tweedles, you're stuck with me, and I'm stuck with you. You go home, and I'll stay here and come back later."

Mom says to me, "What is he doing with his foot?"

"I don't know."

He looks at Mom, and says, "Tweets, we have to get this started, or Bud will get mad."

I can feel his nervousness.

The doorbell rings, it's Dee. I open the door and say, "He is acting very strange, not making sense."

She rushes to the bed, and says, "Hi, Mr. Weasley, how are you?"

He doesn't respond, but his eyes become huge and he looks around.

Mom says to him, "Okay Dick, we are going to Babe's, we'll be back later."

The cold air pierces my skin as we walk across the gravel road to the neighbors. It's great to be in a new place. The card game takes several hours to complete. Mom and I stay after most all of the other women are gone. We are not ready to head back to The Scene. Mom continues to complain, "He is so demanding. He always needs something."

Babe replies, "That's his way of communicating with you."

"Why doesn't he just talk?" I ask.

Babe says, "He doesn't know what to say, but I promise you, every time he calls you to the bed he wants to say something."

We walk in the front door at 5:45 p.m. Normally, I come in from the garage, so this is my first time walking in and seeing the picture everyone else does. It is a bit of a shock; the warm entry at the door quickly becomes fear and sadness at The Scene.

Dee says, "He slept almost the whole time. He just woke up not too long ago."

She then says to Mom, "Where is your other home?"

Mom responds, "What do you mean?"

"He keeps saying he wants to go to his second home. Where is it?"

"We don't have another home. This is our only home."

I walk up to the bed, and say, "Hi Dad, what's up?"

"I want to go home."

"You are home."

"Come on Skeets, our other home, let's go."

"You mean in Arizona? We sold it, remember?"

His voice gets louder, "No, my second home. Come on, Molly let's go. You can drive. Go get Mom."

"Dad, we are home. Mom is right here."

"No Molls, our other home. They are having a party and everyone is there. Now Molly, please get Mom, we have to go."

Mom walks over, "What is it Richard?"

His eyes rise, and shine beyond his view. He says, "I saw our new home and it is beautiful."

"Where is it?" she asks.

He whispers, "In the clouds."

Mom looks at me with a *holy shit* kind of grin.

"Tweets, Tweets, please, we have to go," he hollers. "There is a party. They are waiting for us. Let's go."

His arm extends out into the air and his fingers form together in a grabbing motion. He sees something that is elevating his soul.

Mom says to him, "I love you."

Without hesitation, he replies, "I love you too, but I'd love you more if you got in the bed."

His hand is reaching out constantly. It seems his eyes are becoming bluer, eclipsing the white.

Mom asks him, "Dick, what do you see?"

He answers softly, "A wedding reception."

Mom questions, "A wedding reception? Who is there?"

His hand reaches higher, and his eyes widen even more, "Moses and Elijah."

I run to the kitchen for some space. I feel faint. For a few moments I pace back and forth, and then look back out at The Scene.

Mom's mouth is open. She is trying to talk, but her lips are frozen. Dee is sitting in the chair with her hands folded, mumbling a prayer.

Things are definitely different – better, stranger – not scary anymore.

Mom yells, "Molly, Dad wants us to pray."

I take each of my parents' hands and we form our ring. He says, "Dear God, please put me at the top of your list. Please God, give me forgiveness. Please God, please, take care of my beautiful family."

His words become uncertain, soft, and jumbled together. I'm crying so hard I can barely breathe. The phone rings and Mom goes to answer it. She is hysterical; trying to tell whomever it is that she thinks this is the end. Dee is crying as well. I am high on the feeling of peace that engulfs me. His soul is lighter.

Mom hangs up the phone and says, "That was Leslie. She is going to get here as soon as she can, but she has her class tonight."

I say, "You need to call the kids."

Mom replies, "Go get my cell phone, and call Claire. I will call Curtis."

I run to the laundry room with the phone. As I wait for Claire to answer, I am figuring out what I am supposed to say. I don't know if this is the end, or just another stage to get there. She finally answers, "Hello."

"Hi Claire, it's Molly, I think Dad is really close. He is saying weird things, and I think this could be it."

In a somber tone, the same as always, she asks, "Well, what is he saying?"

"He said he saw Moses and Elijah and then he prayed this crazy prayer. He is acting weird, and I just wanted to let you know."

"Okay, well, I'm at work, and they don't like it when I have personal issues, but I will try to get there as soon as I can."

I walk back into the room. Dad's arm is high in the air trying to catch something. I say to Dee, "Do you know what is going on?"

She looks directly at me, and says, "The Devil and the Lord are fighting for his soul, but today the Lord is winning. Your father sees his new home and he is amazed by its beauty."

"Have you seen this before?"

"No, never, but I have read about it. He sees Heaven right now and he wants to go."

I walk back over to his side, "Hi Dad, what is going on?"

He replies, "I left money on the bar, we have to get it."

I hear the front door open. It's Lynn. I run over and fall into her arms, saying, "I think this is it."

She takes a deep breath, "I know. Leslie just called me. She can't get out of class. She told me to tell you, she will be here as soon as she can. How is he?"

She makes her way to The Scene, "Hi Dick, how are you?"

He turns, but looks through her, and does not say anything.

He calls out, "Molly, we have to get the truck out of the ditch before the cops get here."

A few minutes have gone by, his mouth is locked open and his intense blue eyes are still wide, looking at something in the distance. His hand floats in front of him and his fingers deliberately grab the air. He whispers, "We need to go to our new home. They are waiting for us. There is a party. Please, go get Mom."

"Dad, you go ahead, we will follow you."

"I don't understand why you are being so difficult, Skeeters. Now we need to go home together, in the car. You can drive, Skeeters. Go get Mom."

Mom and Lynn move to the bed. His eyes open even wider and look up at the ceiling. Mom asks, "What do you see, Richard?"

His hand reaches higher.

"Moses," he mumbles.

His fingers continue to caress the air.

"But I don't have a good suit," he laments.

Mom replies, "You have a beautiful suit."

"It's not the right kind."

Mom looks at me and says, "Is he talking about his funeral?"

"I don't think that's what he means," I answer.

Lynn says, "I don't think so either."

My phone rings, it's Kate. She asks, "What's going on?"

"Dad is acting very weird. We think this could be it."

"Let me talk to him."

I put the phone to his ear and say, "Dad, it's Kate."

He says, "Hi, Katie."

"Yes," he answers a question. I'm not sure what she told him, but he then says, "Okay, I love you too, Katie."

I put the phone back up to my ear as I walk into the kitchen. I ask, "What happened?"

"I asked him if he accepted Jesus Christ as his lord and savior and he said yes."

I hang up the phone feeling disoriented. I fall to my knees, sobbing.

"Oh Molly!" Mom yells, and runs in, sheltering me with her arms. She picks me up off the floor and says, "It's okay, Molls."

"I know, Mom, I know."

We sit together, not moving. He cries out, "Come on Ma, let's go home. Please take me home."

Mom gets up and walks over to him, "Richard, you can go. I will be right behind you."

Lynn and I proceed to The Scene, as he yells, "Curtis, get down! Turn the wheel. Turn the wheel! Hit the break. Stop, stop!"

I feel drunk. What is really happening here?

He says, "Molly, please, I'm begging you to take me home."

"Okay Dad, let's go."

"Where is your mom?"

Mom replies, "I'm going to be right behind you."

He screams out, "Tweedles, we have this beautiful home, please, let's go. Please, take me home."

His arm never comes down, constantly trying to reach something off in the distance. He says, "Come on Molly, you can drive."

"Okay, Dad."

His hand falls down and extends toward me as he says, "Here's the keys, let's go."

I grab the keys of air from his hand, "Okay, I'm starting it up."

"Where is your mom? You need to get Mom?"

I make eye contact with him and say, "Dad, she will be right behind us. She is fine. We are going to go."

"Okay, let's go Skeeters."

My hands are shaped as though I'm steering the wheel. I pretend to drive him home and it doesn't feel like an imaginary thing, but something more real than I've ever experienced.

"Okay, we are home. Here we are."

"Open the garage door," he eagerly replies.

"Okay, it's open."

"No, it won't open. Come on Molly, open the door."

"Dad it's opening right now."

He pauses for a moment. Then in an anxious tone, he asks, "Where is your mom?"

"She is right behind us, Dad."

"No, the garage door won't open until she gets here. Now, go get your mom. I want to go home."

He gets quiet, his breathing slows as he calms, and then falls asleep.

Lynn says, "He is as peaceful as I've ever seen him. What a difference from the other night."

She then says, "You guys are running on pure adrenalin. Soon you will have a huge void, then you will resume."

Being within the ropes is not easy: making sure he is equipped for the holes to come, making sure he is physically and mentally prepared. Guiding him down these long and hilly fairways is tiresome. As much as I want this round to be over, as difficult as it is, I know this will be the last time I carry his bag, and I will mourn these yards we tread together.

Claire comes through the door. She asks, "How is he?"

"He just finally fell asleep," I reply.

For about a half hour, Claire and I sit at his bedside, with Mom and Lynn just a few feet away. The silence is soothing.

Claire says, "He is really out."

"Yeah, I'm sorry, when I called you things were crazy. I can't believe how calm he is."

"You didn't know, it's okay," she says.

We sit together at our father's deathbed, as he fades away, back into holiness.

Are we bonding, somehow?

Another thirty minutes go by and Claire says, "I have to go."

She kisses his forehead, "It's Claire, Dad. I love you."

*

I am staring into the refrigerator, dazed with exhaustion, when I hear his voice, "Ma, get me some ice cream."

I shout out, "I got it."

I get his ice cream quickly because I am anxious to see what happens. I move him forward to feed him.

"How do you feel?" I ask.

"Thirsty."

"This will help," I say, putting the spoon to his lips.

He barely opens his mouth, but easily lets the ice cream slide in. He savors the coolness of the sweet, milky substance as he swooshes it around. He is taking forever, but I am okay with it this time. His eyes open really big; he looks at me knowingly. I believe the meaning of life may spill off his lips.

"Sip of pop, Skeets," he finally says.

"Sip of pop, my ass," I mutter as I turn to the table to get his glass.

He sips it as strongly as he can. He is thirsty from his journey.

Leslie walks in the door and asks, "What's going on? How is he doing?"

She walks to the bed and opens her bag. She checks his heart with a stethoscope. She says, "His heart rate is a bit low."

His hand reaches out. Leslie says to him, "How do you feel, Dick?"

He doesn't respond, but his eyes are bigger than I thought possible.

Headlights shine in through the window. Mom says, "Who is that now?"

"Zack," Dad replies.

Lynn looks out the window and says, "It is Zack. Dick, how did you know that?"

No response, for he is starting to see visions again. His eyes are on the ceiling and his arm is reaching toward it.

Zack walks through the door and asks, "Is everything okay?"

Lynn responds, "Yeah, Leslie just got here."

"Is that you, Zack?" Dad says.

Zack has already perceived that something is different as he approaches, "Hey Weasel."

We are all close in a circle around The Scene in the most peaceful silence possible. Dad stares at the ceiling. His hand is high, still grabbing. I look at Leslie, and ask, "What is he doing?"

She replies, "He is reaching for Heaven."

"Really?"

She nods her head and says, "Yeah, my dad did it right before. I think we are very close."

"You do?" Mom says.

Leslie smiles as she watches him, "He sees Heaven, it's

near, and he wants to go. He is trying to grab hold of it."

I see Zack's face and I'm guessing mine looks about the same—*deer in the headlights.*

At least thirty minutes have gone by and nobody has said a word. We only gaze at him, feeling the true serenity of the power overtaking the room.

He begins to get restless, and says, "Let's go home."

Mom replies, "Richard, you can go, and we will be right behind you."

"Oh, you say that. Why do you have to be such a donkey nuts? Why can't we just go home?"

I should pray now, I should say something.

"Why don't we say a prayer?" I suggest.

He says, "No, I don't want to. Let's go home."

My stomach is twisted into a knot. I am disappointed. Mom says, "Richard, we are going to pray."

Everyone grabs hands around the bed. I say, "Dear God, please watch over my father and guide him in your direction. Please, give him the strength to go with you and—"

I choke up, start coughing, and can't get the words out, until finally a feeble *Amen* rolls off my tongue The *Amen* passes from everyone else's lips. Tears are running down my face, I sit down. Zack, now in a chair behind me, puts his hand on my shoulder, and I lean back into his chest. Mom, Lynn, and Leslie are huddled around watching Dad, trying to understand the moment. All of a sudden, he points down and mumbles something. Mom asks him, "What did you say, Richard?"

He hollers, "Oh, you know Tweets, that black lab we had, Becker"

"You see Becker?" I ask.

"Yeah, he is right over there. He wants us to come home."

Rebecca, the Christian, gave me Becker as a puppy. I left him home when I moved away. He was Dad's dog anyway. Dad always said he hoped Becker would outlive him because it would be too hard to put him down. This wish was destroyed just months ago, the day after Thanksgiving, when Becker lay in his spot, and the vet injected forever rest.

Dad screams, "Watch out! Watch out! Hit the ditch!"

Mom asks, "Is there someone with you?"

"I wish there was," his hand extends out again.

He whispers, "Thanks for the wonderful life, Tweets. I want you to take me to Heaven. Come on, Tweets. Let's go, let's go."

"You can go, Richard. You can go."

I feel like I am floating.

He is quiet and completely hypnotized by the image beyond our existence.

Zack finally says, "I think I'm going to head out."

Lynn replies, "I will be right behind you."

Zack stops at the door and turns around to take one final look. He is captured by the essence of what he sees, and he stands there, frozen. Another twenty minutes go by before Lynn says, "We have to go."

She passes Zack's statue, and he follows her out the door.

It's almost eleven o'clock. I have a feeling it's going to be a night like no other. I need a shower and a smoke to prepare. I receive a text from Kate:

Why do I love this man so much when he mistreated us so much?

Good question.

Dad says to Mom, "I love you so much, let's just go home. I will show you my love and affection. I promise."

He tilts his head at Mom, and whispers, "I don't understand why you and Molly never were close."

Everyone is quiet.

His head cocks up to Leslie, "Leslie, can I ask you a favor?"

"Sure, Dick."

"Will you take care of my wife?"

She smiles and touches his shoulder, "Of course."

Empty describes me. Sadness engulfs me. Distance is more than just yards.

*

He is trying to start the mower with his hands. He makes a pulling motion and says, "Crank it up, Molls. Crank it up. Push the button to start the machine."

He grabs my hand and starts making a circular motion, "Get the key."

I pretend to find the key in the bed and act as though I'm starting something up. He yells, "Come on, Molly. It won't go."

"What, Dad?"

Full of frustration, he responds, "The mower. Now take these two wires and put them together."

I put my hands in front of him and motion my fingers to display that I am putting two wires together. He watches me closely and soon shouts, “Now pull the lever.”

“Okay Dad, we are good. It’s all good.”

His foot begins to move. He says, “I can’t reach the pedal. Please help me, Molly. Come on Molly, why won’t it go?”

He calms down suddenly as he reaches out into the air. His eyes become wide, looking up and all around.

*

It is a few minutes until 1:00 a.m. He screams out, “Let’s go home. Please, let’s go home.”

I can’t take my eyes off of him. He calms down for a moment, but soon yells out, “Becker! Come on Ma, Becker is right there, let’s go home.”

I respond, “Dad, you can go now and give Becker a kiss for me.”

His eyes get huge, the biggest so far, as he looks right at me and says, “Molly, I’m ready to go. I love you Molly you are my daughter. Help me go. Help me go, please.”

Within moments, his heartwarming words turn into frightened screams, “Turn the wheel hard! Harder, harder, watch out! Curtis, Curtis!”

I say with a stern voice, “Dad, Dad, calm down it’s okay.”

He quiets down and after a long pause he whispers, “I want my—”, but we can’t understand anymore. He then tries again, “I want my—”

Mom asks him, “What, what do you want, Dick?”

He shouts out at the top of his lungs, “I want my pop!”

Leslie yells out, giggling, “He wants his pop.”

Mom says, “Oh Dick, you are unbelievable

sometimes."

He takes a sip and blurts out, "Let's go home!"

Mom replies, "Okay Richard, you go ahead, and I'll be right behind you. I'll be home later."

He says, "Work, work, work, you are going to kill yourself."

Leslie says, "You got your second wind."

He replies, "I'd like to get my first wind, but that's out of the question."

Mom is lying down on the mattress. Leslie and I are up, glued to The Scene.

He says to me, "Come on Molly, get Mom, and let's go home."

I respond deliberately as though I am talking to a two year old, "Dad, you have to go first, and Mom will come later."

He yells back at me, "Molly, get in the car."

"Dad, we have to follow you in the other car."

"No, you can drive. Now start the car."

"Okay Dad, here we go."

I am really going to make it work this time. I'm going to get him home. I am driving the car, "We are going now. We're on our way, Dad."

I allow some time to go by and then say, "Okay, we are home, but I have to drop you off and come back later."

"Okay, Skeets, open the garage door."

Oh shit, him and the damn garage door.

"Okay, it's open."

He, without any hesitation responds, "Where is your

mom?"

"She is right behind us."

"Come on Molly. Why won't the garage door open? Please let's go home."

I can't argue this situation anymore. He is as stubborn as he always was. I say, "Dad, you can go, and Mom will be right behind you."

With a soft, disappointed voice he says, "Okay Skeeters, thanks for your assistance."

He grabs my hand, hypnotized by it. He reminds me of a baby again, as he stares and plays with my fingers. Twenty minutes go by without a sound while he still holds my hand. He finally unclenches his fingers from mine and begins to settle down. He is about to fall asleep. Leslie gets up and moves to a couch, saying, "We need to take advantage of this moment."

She is right. I snuggle into the other couch, and thank the Lord for the peacefulness I see in my father.

"Judy, Judy," he screams out.

I just fell asleep.

He shouts, "Tweedy, are you ready to go home?"

My eyes are open now but my head pushes deep into the pillow, trying to remove myself from his voice. He screams, "Judy, Claire, Bridges…Bridges!"

And then, "Molly, Molly!"

I rise, and wobble over my blanket to The Scene, "Yeah, Dad?"

He demands, "Go get your mom, so we can go home."

He wants to go home and asks for my help. Home is the place we are when we have no other place to be. It is the most comfortable place we know. During a lifetime how many times does a person say, 'I want to go home'?

His pupils are even bigger than before. He is on his way to greatness with those bright blue eyes. He is interested in something beyond the ceiling.

Mom whispers, "What does he see?"

I reply, "I don't know, but he is going crazy."

His arm reaches the highest I've seen. He yells out with a bit of a stutter, "Is that my mother?"

He pauses, leans forward sitting completely upright, and yells, "Holy shit!"

His face stunned as he slowly moves his lips, "That is my mom."

I look at Leslie and say, "Did he just see his own mother?"

"Appears so."

Mom gets up from the mattress, "What do you see, Richard?"

He is captivated with what's before him.

Mom tries once more, "What do you see?"

His voice is soft, but confident, "Jesus."

"Jesus? Where is he at?" I exclaim.

"Five feet away," he whispers as his arm extends even farther. His hand and fingers move frantically through the air. My whole body tingles. I imagine white clouds, Dad here and Jesus there, but only Dad can really see him.

He turns to Mom, "I'm so sorry. I'm ready to go."

She sighs from exhaustion as she says, "It is okay, Richard, you can go."

Of all the holes played thus far, today the sun shines the brightest. His shots have landed on the plush fairway. He can even see the eighteenth hole in the distance, and the magnificent clubhouse sitting behind the green. He knows his new home awaits him.

Mom and Leslie, each wrapped in a blanket, have their heads resting on their hands, leaning on the rails.

Suddenly he jerks up and yells, "Stop! Stop! Straight ahead! Watch out Curtis! Hit the brake!"

Within seconds he is calm and reaching again as if he has never seen anything so beautiful. He starts to wrestle around. He shouts out, "Come on Ma, we are all ready to go, and you're the last one to leave."

I have positioned myself against the rail on the other side of the bed from Mom and Leslie. From here I can see the table of essentials needed for our wait: creams, toothpaste, hairbrush, gauze, toilet paper, spray bottles. It's basically the combination between a bathroom and a hospital room.

The cancer-cleaning bottle is hurting my eyes.

I don't understand its purpose; it only cleans, it does not heal. Seems like a half-ass job to me.

I turn my attention back to him. He asks, "Leslie, are you in favor of leaving?"

She shines a smile upon him and says, "I think it would be a good thing."

He, in a slow motion way turns to me and says, "What about you, Skeeters?"

His eyes are full of wonder as he reaches out beyond me. I lean in and say, "Dad, I promise you can go, it will be all right."

It's easy to sin if you can get away with it, but for how long? Even if you never have to face the ones you hurt, you still have to face yourself. You can wait until the end, but before it's over you will find yourself on the toughest hole, with unplayable shots, admitting to penalties, and seeing the green ahead, but not having the energy to get there.

It's almost 5:00 a.m., when he shouts, "Here comes the train."

He recognizes something and his eyes go straight up. He says, "Do you still bowl?"

His hand moves toward his mouth and he takes a bite of air. Mom asks him, "What are you eating?"

"Three pieces of fish."

"Where are you?"

He refuses her question this time. He is involved with his, no longer lonely, voyage. He points in the distance and says, "Look at the size of that turd. That turd has to be a mile long."

We laugh so hard that Mom can't catch her breath.

He yells, "It's just a turd, Tweets, that's all."

We are still giggling when he says, "Are we staying overnight again? You can, but I'm gonna' go home. Becker, I'm coming home, boy."

Within a few moments he is making the eating motion again. I ask him, "What are you eating?"

"A strawberry melt, but I don't want it, it's too smooshie," he says, as he hands me a palm of air.

He looks straight at Leslie and says, "Now, I'll bet you a hundred dollar bill that come nine we will be sitting on our ass."

She replies, "You think so?"

"I know so, Les, but I just don't understand why we

can't go home."

Mom says, "Here we go again."

He is furious, yelling in his loudest voice, "Son of a bitch! We have this beautiful home and you won't go."

I need a break. I don't want to have this conversation anymore.

I get up and head to the couch. He screams, "Molly, are we gonna' go home? You drive, I have a headache."

I stop in my tracks, "*You* have a headache? Shit, what do I have?"

"Come on Molls, let's go home. Please, let's just go home."

I continue to the couch and lie down.

A few minutes later he screams, "Hit the break! Stop! Stop! Stop!"

I get up and hobble back to the chair. I put this chair beside the bed about ten hours ago. I have sat in it, lain in it, laughed, and cried in it. I spent almost the entire night in it. I'm stuck in it. Even though I am on the other side of the rails, I too, am captive.

He calls out, "Molly, Molly, Daisy is here!"

I yell back, "Daisy?"

Daisy was our first dog. She was a mean little shit.

"Molly, do you see Daisy?"

"No, but, who else do you see, Dad?"

"I'm not sure, I don't know their names."

His arm is reaching high and his eyes widen again.

I say, "I have to lie down and close my eyes. I love you, Dad. Go to sleep now."

I lean down and kiss his forehead.

It is 5:37 a.m., as I lie down to finally sleep.

At 6:02 a.m. he screams out, "Skeeters, would you please come here."

Leslie is at the bed, "Molly, your father wants you."

I teeter upright, "Okay Dad, what's up?"

I curl up in the chair, lay my head on the rails, and watch him.

Happiness covers him. The amazement in his eyes tells me there is too much to see and learn. The dazzling glare of an ocean blue lightens the room. No eyes shine that bright. A powerful essence is causing them to glow.

He whispers, "She's gonna' leave me. Come on, Molls, come on, get your mom."

"Dad, I promise you, she will not leave you. She will be right behind you."

A few minutes go by. He screams out, "Curtis! Oh shit! Claire! We are going to get in trouble if the cops come. Stop! Stop! Stop the car! Jesus Christ, stop the car!"

He is the most terrified I've seen him so far. He hollers out, "Okay Ma, get my ID and my bank card and put it away for me, I'm going home."

I am back on the couch when he calls me, "Molly, would you come here for a moment please?"

I run to his side, and he says, "Press this button."

Shortly after, he cries, "Come on Skeets, press it again, we have to get this working."

His foot is moving up and down as though it was pushing a pedal on a piano.

I remain silent to see what he does next.

His eyes are now really big as his arm reaches out. I say to him, "Grab his hand, Dad. God is ready for you, go ahead."

His fingers caress my face. He examines my features, "Hi, you are my daughter."

"Hi, you are my father," my heart softens. "Now close your eyes and go to sleep and I will see you in Heaven."

I gently kiss him and float back to the couch as dawn creeps through the window. My hands fold, "Please Lord, let him sleep. Let us all just sleep."

Day 32

A loud thumping opens my eyes. I walk to the door, fumble to open it, and see Heather standing there.

"Rough night?" she asks.

"Crazy."

I head back to the couch and fall into it.

She asks, "What happened?"

Mom is lying on the floor. She raises her head; her hair is a mess.

Heather sees her and says, "Oh my God! What happened?"

"He saw some things," Mom replies. "We were up all night. We thought, for sure—"

"What kind of things?" Heather asks.

Mom yawns, "Moses and Elijah. I don't know, you ask him."

Heather approaches Dad, "How was your night?"

He looks up at her and says, "Everybody is going to town to get on the boat. There is going to be a big party."

Mom gets up from the air mattress, "Richard, what are you talking about?"

With confidence, he says, "I know what I'm gonna' do. I don't care what you do."

I say to Heather, "This has been going on since yesterday afternoon. It started, with the mower thing. Then we left, and when we got back, he was saying and seeing crazy stuff. He fell asleep a couple times, but not for long, and when he woke up, I don't know, he said a lot of things."

"What do you mean?" Heather asks.

"The things he said and saw," I reply.

Mom continues to tell the story, as Heather cleans Dad's tumor.

"What time is it anyway?" I ask.

"It's nine on the dot," Heather answers.

Leslie pops up and says, "You were right, Dick, it is nine, and we are sitting on our asses."

Everyone laughs as we continue to discuss the night.

"His heart rate is much slower," Heather says.

She then asks, "When is the last time he ate?"

Mom replies, "He had breakfast and lunch yesterday, and some ice cream last night."

"I'll come back around noon with the hospice chaplain," Heather explains. "It sounds like he is having some spiritual issues, and I think our chaplain could help. He is very close. You may want to call loved ones and let them know."

Mom goes into the bedroom with the phone.

She soon returns, "Everyone is going to be here soon."

As she brushes Dad's hair she says, "Richard, your sister is coming."

I can tell he is about to get another glimpse of Heaven, as his arm and eyes begin the process. Mom notices the transformation too, and asks him, "What do you see Richard?"

His voice is content, he says, "They're golfing."

"Who?" Mom questions.

"Eli Mertens."

"Eli Mertens. Who else?"

His hand is the highest it has been, but his replies have ended because he is too amused by what he sees.

"Eli Mertens died over twenty-five years ago. He was another of Dad's best friends," Mom comments.

*

It is a few minutes after 11:00 a.m., and many spectators surround The Scene.

He is back on his mission, saying, "Come on Molls, get in the car, let's go home."

I'm trying to think of the perfect response.

He hollers, "You can drive, and I'll ride along to keep you company."

"Okay, Dad."

We go through the whole motion just like before.

"Open the garage door. The garage door won't open. Where is your mom? Mom, Ma."

"Dad, okay, we will go home, but here is the deal—"

"God dammit, no more deals. Please just let me go home."

Grandma grabs his hand and says, “His arms are open for you, Richard.”

“I don’t want to fall,” he cries out.

She responds, “God won’t let you fall, he will catch you.”

He is reaching strongly now. His energy has increased, trying to grab his way to freedom. We all watch his motions, trying to understand. I’m the closest to him, holding his hand. Aunt Susan, Grandma, and Aunt Judy sit around the silver rails. Leslie and Mom are in the background. Bridgett holds baby Hunter, facing the foot of the bed. We are engrossed by his every action.

“Molly, help me crank it up.”

I begin to twist my hand in a circular motion, and he screams, “More, more, come on, Molls, turn the key. Turn the key!”

“Where are you going?” I shout.

“To Hell and back!” he screams.

We are all taken back by his comment.

“Lost the key, where is the key, Molly?”

Aunt Susan decides to play along. “Here it is,” she says, as her finger comes my way.

“Thank you,” I reply, making a grabbing motion.

“Okay Skeeters, help me get this mower going.”

Once again, I play his routine.

“The battery must be dead,” he shouts.

“No Dad, it's fine.”

“Start it up, Molls.”

I try, but he soon cries out, “Bud is gonna’ get mad. We

need to get this going. Please Molly, help me reach the pedal."

His foot begins to twitch.

"Please Molls, push me up to the pedal."

I turn to Mom, and say, "You need to call Bud and have him come over, now."

Dad cries, "Come on Skeeters, please take me home. Everyone has a different opinion, but it's time we go home."

He calms down quickly, and appears to have another vision.

He is in radiance again. He sees the beauty of innocence and seeks it for himself.

"Who is on the roof?" he asks.

Mom walks to his side to get a better look at the way his eyes are moving. She asks him, "What do you see, Richard?"

"There is someone on the roof."

"The roof?"

"Yeah Tweets, there is someone on the roof. Up there, on the roof, who is it?"

He points to the ceiling, "Up there, Tweets, he is painting."

"Painting? Who is painting?"

"The painter, up there. He is on the roof."

"Do you know who the painter is, Richard?"

He sighs, "Yeah."

"Who is it?"

His hand reaches high in the air and his fingers make a grabbing motion. He whispers, "Leslie's father."

I turn to Leslie. Her face is white, dazed by what she heard.

I ask her, "Did he know your father?"

In a state of confusion, she responds, "No, not at all."

"Did you ever tell him about your dad?"

She shakes her head, "No. I never talked to him about my father. He never knew him. When he died, I didn't even know you guys yet."

She wipes her eye with a balled up tissue, and smiles, "But he was a painter."

Mom, with a bit of apprehension, turns to her, "He was?"

"I was very young. That's what he did when I was a kid, but I have no idea how Dick would know that."

She approaches the bed, and asks, "Dick, can you hear me?"

His head turns toward her. With sparkling eyes he calmly whispers, "It's all right, everything is fine. I promise you, everything is just fine. Now finish your game so I can get this mower back to the shed."

Bud walks through the door.

"Oh my God, perfect timing," I say, as he walks up to the bed.

"Hi Dick. It's Bud."

Dad turns to Bud and looks as though he is going to cry. After a calm pause he says, "I'm so sorry Bud, but I can't get it fixed."

"It is okay, Dick. It's all right."

"But we need to get it back to the barn."

Bud, trying to ease his worry responds, "The boys took care of it. It's already there. Everything is going really well, you don't need to worry about anything."

Dad becomes quiet and still.

I ask Bud, "Do you know of an incident on the seventeenth green where a mower got stuck?"

Bud says, "Yeah, it was right when your dad quit working. He thought the mower was stuck and he called Luke out to help him. Luke said there was nothing wrong with the mower at all. He realized, your dad's foot gave out and he didn't have the strength to push the pedal."

We had no idea why he quit, he never told anyone. Dad maintained the grass for over twenty-five years. The golf course was all he knew. He would get up, mow it, run home, take a shower, then go out and play on it. At the end of the day he would sit on the deck and watch the sun set over it. Nobody was closer to the fairways than him.

We all sit, stunned.

Dad says, "Hey Bud, how many years has the golf course been open?"

"Oh, about forty-seven, forty-eight years."

I blurt out, "I bet all the money in the world it's forty-seven."

Bridgett whispers, "I just got the chills."

Bud grabs Dad's hand and says, "I have to go Dick. I have a guy waiting for me at the clubhouse. I want to thank you for all your help, and I'll make sure the boys take care of everything. You don't need to worry."

Dad looks up at him, "Okay Bud, thanks for stopping by."

Bud closes the door, leaving us in a dream. Our minds are consumed with what we can't explain.

"I see a box," Dad says.

I reply, "A box? What does it look like?"

"It's just a box, Molly."

"Well, does it have anything on it?"

"There is a number on it."

I'm scared to ask, but do anyway, "A number, really what is the number?"

"Oh Molly, it's just forty-eight."

I look at Aunt Susan, as she shrugs her shoulders and says, "Close enough."

"Are we at our house?" Dad asks.

Mom replies, "Yes we are."

"Hey Ma, I want to sit here and watch Dick Tracy."

"Dick Tracy? You never watched Dick Tracy."

Aunt Judy pipes up says, "Oh yes, he did. When he was a boy it was his favorite thing."

This knowledge of childhood joy is soothing.

Heather arrives with the chaplain. They walk up to the bed, and Heather says, "Richard, this is Brett, he is our hospice chaplain."

"Hi there, Richard. You have a lot of people here today with you," the chaplain says.

"Yeah, they are here for the wedding."

"A wedding? Who is getting married?"

"I'm not sure, but there is going to be a big party," Dad replies.

His eyes enlarge and he drifts into beauty again.

The chaplain asks him, "Do you mind if we say a prayer?"

Dad responds, "Okay."

His arm reaches out and caresses the air with his fingers. I lay my hand on his shoulder, as all the hands in the room link. It is our biggest circle so far. We bow our heads and expect the chaplain to begin, but it is Dad who speaks.

His voice is soft, pleading, as he prays, "Dear God, please forgive me of my sins, and bless my family, and the people in California."

He stutters, but continues to recite his final hopes. As his tone becomes weaker, he mumbles, "Thank you Lord, for all your charity, and please help out all the old people who are sick."

Our cries and sniffles become louder, as he says, "Amen."

We all repeat, "Amen."

His eyes open wide, and his finger extends toward the ceiling. He yells out, "Now, if you want to be a good golfer, watch that lady over there. Even though she is ninety-one she will knock your dick straight."

The room erupts with laughter. Aunt Judy falls off of her chair. Heather and the chaplain run to help her, but they can't stop laughing and struggle with the simple task.

Once everyone has calmed down, the chaplain says, "Now, that is one I've never heard."

Everyone breaks away from The Scene, chuckling.

Heather says, "I'm going to put in the catheter now."

I walk toward the kitchen, puzzling over these mystical

moments. The chaplain approaches me and says, "He is very interesting."

I ask him, "What exactly is going on?"

He replies, "What is going on here is very real. He sees Heaven and is reaching out for it. The wedding reception is his celebration. It is to welcome him. He sees them preparing for it. Those people he sees are waiting for his arrival, and everyone here today is waiting for his departure. We let go of one hand, and they will grab the other. He will not be alone, but he is scared he will be. He doesn't want to go by himself. He still doesn't have complete faith that he will be okay. You need to reinforce his confidence. Tell him it is okay to go and he doesn't need your mother. Convince him she needs to stay at this time, but will soon be behind him."

I have no response. I just stare at him, waiting for more. He continues, "Honestly, I have never been more amazed by a patient. Heather has kept me informed. Your dad is already a rare case because he can't have sedative drugs. By this time in the process for most, either the symptoms are so bad, or they are on so much medication that this could not be possible. Now, here in his presence, I can feel the harmony in the air. It is overwhelming. You are very blessed as a family."

On cue, Dad's voice calls, "Come on Ma, let's go home."

Heather is the only one at The Scene, trying to calm him down. The rest of us stand in the dining room, watching the two of them together. Dad says to her, "It's been a long day, and it's been a long night. I will probably pass, but I will see you again, soon."

Heather walks toward me, tears running down her face. She says, "It is close. You need to call the other kids and let them know."

She continues, "Don't forget, you can call Courtney at any time tonight. I will let her know the status when I leave."

I must look dazed. She embraces me, and I hug her tightly.

"Come on Ma, it's time to go home," Dad cries out.

The chaplain says, "Come on, let's go tell him it's okay."

Like a herd of sheep, we assemble around the bed.

"Let's go, Ma. Come on. We have to go."

Bridgett is the first to respond to his plea, "Tweedy has to stay, Grandpa. She has some things to do before she can go, but she will be fine. You go ahead, and she will be right behind you."

"Richard, everything is going to be fine," Mom grabs his hand. "You need to go now, it's your time. When my time comes, I will follow."

Grandma puts her hand on top of Mom's, on top of Dad's, and says, "Richard you need to go and be with the Lord. He is calling you."

Tears fill the room again.

Heather says, "We are leaving now, Richard. I will see you soon."

Dad is too busy reaching for the glory he sees, to give a response.

The chaplain puts his arm around me, and says, "You are in the middle of a miracle. Savor it, and good luck."

Dad is in a reaching frenzy, as everyone else prepares to leave.

"I'm ready to go. Where is my hat?" Dad yells out.

sleep."

She turns to me and says, "I am going to go lie down."

She disappears into the hall.

My heavy eyes fall into darkness as I doze off for a brief instant, until he cries, "Come on, Ma."

His shirt is on the floor. I approach the bed and notice something in his hand. I recognize the bandage from his tumor.

"Oh no!" I scream out, "Dad, what are you doing?"

His hands are rapid and his fingers are picking at everything on him and around him, while I try to replace the bandage.

I decide to call hospice, to see if there is anything I can do to calm not only him but also me. Courtney is on the other end of the line, as I describe the situation.

"He is agitated right now, and beginning the picking stage," she explains.

Another stage? I thought this was it.

I rub his cheek, trying to help the drops dissolve. "Dad, this will calm you down and then you need to go to sleep. Please Dad, try to go to sleep."

He doesn't respond. He is busy picking fuzz from the blanket, but seemingly unaware of his new habit. The next hour is childish, he throws his shirt on the floor and I replace it, repeatedly. I watch him pull it off, and I am stupid enough to keep allowing it. After another hour, he finally calms down. I think he may even be asleep.

*

The opening of the door has become a familiar alarm. I open my eyes to see Babe and Henry walk in. I thought it must be the next day, but it's dark outside. Babe's hands are tight in the pockets of her black leather coat as she walks to The Scene. Her arms are tense from the cold air outside.

Mom says, "He is finally asleep. He's been up for more than twenty-four hours!"

Babe sits at the table, listening to our story of the past day, flipping through the hospice book. She says, "This is interesting. Has he talked about his funeral?"

"No, he hasn't done that yet," Mom answers.

"I think he missed that stage," I add.

Babe replies, "You mean he is past it?"

I reply, "I don't know? What stage is it?"

She looks down at the book and replies, "Forty-seven."

I respond with confusion, "Forty-seven? What?"

She points to the page and says once more, "Forty-seven."

I ask, "What does that mean? Are you being a smart ass?"

Her finger directly hits the bottom of the page, as her voice becomes louder, "It's on page forty-seven. Isn't that what you asked?"

Mom interrupts, "No, she asked you what stage it was, and you said, forty-seven."

Babe replies, "Because I thought she asked what page and it happens to be page forty-seven."

Day 33

It is afternoon, and there is finally movement from within the rails.

"Ma, Ma, let's go home."

I approach him, and ask, "Hi Dad, how are you?"

"Thirsty."

I grab his glass from the table and put the straw to his mouth. "Dad, do you remember yesterday?"

He gulps with much effort. "Yeah, there was a party, Skeets."

"Do you remember who was here?"

He thinks for a moment, and then answers, "Heather the nurse."

"Yeah, that's right, she was."

"She was changing her outfit."

Puzzled, I ask him, "What was she wearing?"

He softly sighs, "A wedding dress."

"A wedding dress? Are you sure?"

"I don't know if it was her, but everyone was trying on their outfits."

I continue to question him, "Who else was here?"

He thinks for a moment, "A big guy was at the table, waiting for the wedding."

"A big guy, who was it?"

His voice is soft, but confident, "John."

"John? Who is that?"

"He was sitting down at a table reading the book. He needs to get ready for the party."

"Who is John?"

"He is at the banquet, waiting, but the church is beautiful, it's outside. Hey Molls, look."

His hand grabs toward the sky.

"What is it, Dad?"

"The atmosphere is snowy white."

"Like the clouds?"

"Yeah, like the clouds," he whispers.

He is quiet after that, for a while.

"Molly, get me my white robe," he demands.

"You don't have a robe."

"Yes I do, ask your Mother, she will get it."

I yell down the hall, "Hey Mom, does Dad have a robe?"

She yells back, "What? He doesn't have a robe."

"I figured. I didn't think you did. Dad, you don't have a robe."

He whines, "Please, get me my white robe, or I will look goofy."

"Richard, what are you talking about?" Mom, irritated, comes from the hall.

"My robe Ma, get my robe."

"Richard, you don't have a robe."

He is quiet. Mom and I regroup in the kitchen.

Within minutes, his hands are reckless again, reaching, grabbing, and picking. Mom runs to him, picking his shirt off of the floor on her way, "Richard, you need to stop."

"Get my white robe," he shouts.

Mom responds, "You don't have a white robe."

"Tweets, please, I need my white robe."

Mom, now a bit more vocal, says, "Dick, you don't have a robe."

He pauses, in great thought.

In an inquiring voice, he says, "Hey Tweets, the other night at the party there was a little boy. Do you know who he is?"

Mom, baffled, asks, "A little boy, what did he look like?"

"About nine years old, in greasy clothes—grimy little guy."

I walk up to him and ask, "Grimy? Who could that be?"

"I don't know. That's why I'm asking Mom to tell me."

"Richard, I don't know a little boy," Mom says.

"He was bussing the tables at the party. Who is he, Tweets?"

"I don't know, Dick."

"He was at the banquet. I am just asking you to tell me who he is. Everyone is wearing their outfits but him. Please, Tweets, the little boy."

"Richard, I don't know. Now, please keep your shirt on."

Dad wants to be clothed in the attire of everyone else he sees. They made the cut and are robed in purity. There is a guy named John reading a book, while awaiting the wedding. Dad's last hole is near, and his score will soon be counted. Is John the scorekeeper; the one who posts his score?

The neighbors, Jack and Janet, stop by. They stand around the bed having a final chat about golf.

Jack asks Dad, "Who is your favorite golfer, Dick?"

Dad doesn't reply.

We start naming famous golfers. After five or so names are tossed out, Dad interrupts, "You're all wrong, it's Payne Stewart."

"Payne Stewart! You always made fun of his knickers," I say.

His fingers knead the air as he whispers, "He still wears them underneath."

He then asks, "Molls, can I have some ice cream?"

I go and open the freezer.

Underneath? It's strange he chose Payne Stewart. I watched a lot of golf with my dad, and I'm surprised that's his answer. Payne Stewart has been dead for years.

The neighbors are gone. I stand at The Scene feeding him ice cream, when he says, "Molls, put the golf on."

This is the most coherent he has been since Monday

morning, and he is eating, too. He didn't eat for a day, but now his appetite is back.

He is taking his usual amount of time to eat, so I turn to the television. My eyes become huge as I see an image of Payne Stewart on the screen. The words blare from the box, "A look back at Payne Stewart."

I turn to Dad, and say, "How stupid."

He replies, "My crack needs to be rolled."

I can't help but snicker, "I figured you would say something like that."

"Come on Molly, I'm in pain here."

"Mom!"

She shouts from the office, "What?"

"Dick is back, and he needs to be rolled."

The last time we rolled him was Monday morning. I didn't even think about it because he hasn't complained in two days.

Mom walks out, and says, "What's going on now?"

Dad says, "My crack hurts, and my feet are on fire."

Day 34

I walk out to another morning. Mom is at the scene. His silver hair glares off the rails.

This picture will soon only exist in my mind.

"When am I going to get my tumor fixed?"

Mom replies, "Nothing can be done for your tumor, Richard."

"Then, I just want to go and be with the Lord."

*

Today has been quiet, no visitors, and Dad is more peaceful.

"Hey Skeeters, you need to take me to town, to the hair stylist."

"The hair stylist? What hair stylist?"

"I need to get ready. Everyone is waiting. They are all waiting."

"Waiting for what, Dad?"

"The wedding," he whispers.

His eyes flicker and then close.

"Whose wedding, Dad?"

His energy is gone; the visions hinder his body, but strengthen his soul.

After an hour of solitude in the office, I walk out to the living room. Mom hangs up the phone. She says, "Aunt Judy just told me that when they were kids, they lived above a garage that worked on big trucks. She said that Dad and Buck always came home covered in grease, and Grandma Betty would always yell at them for being so 'greasy and grimy'. She said they loved to play in that garage."

Day 35

It's 8:16 a.m., when I wake to bright sun from the bedroom window. I wrap my blanket around me, and head out to the center of entertainment.

Drama, comedy, horror, even news, can be found at The Scene.

Mom is on the mattress, sleeping. Dad is out as well. I creep through the room and down the stairs to my sanctuary.

Nothing makes sense. Why is he still here? Especially after the things he said and saw. Those visions were real; I was there. He should have crossed over by now.

Footsteps thump from above. Tranquility stops, and another ride on this roller coaster begins. I run up the stairs to see what is taking place.

I hear Mom say, "Why do you think that? You shouldn't say that."

Dad's words are not strong enough for me to hear. I get closer, and ask, "What is he saying now?"

"Tell your daughter what you just told me."

Dad is silent and he looks worried about something.

"What is it Dad?"

"I can't go," he blubbers, "because you guys might forget me."

"What? Are you for real? Seriously, this is your biggest worry. God, Dad, figure it out already."

Mom laughs, "You sure are something, Dick."

Aren't there better things to be concerned about on your deathbed? He is the one leaving this infected world, we have to stay and breathe its corrupt air. He's scared that while we try to get by down here, we could forget the fantastic character he portrayed.

Really, Dad?

He's getting a chance to figure it out and he can't. His selfishness is why he lies here, weighed down and crippled with faults he never acknowledged, only buried.

He says he is thirsty, but he keeps spilling with the straw.

I wipe him up, and say, "Okay Dad, here is the straw, suck on it."

The sound of the door opening soothes my tension. Heather says, "Morning. How are we doing this morning?"

I gently take the straw away from his lips and soda appears everywhere. I yell, "Dammit, again?"

As she approaches Heather asks me, "What are you having problems with?"

"For some reason, when he drinks, it spills."

"That happens. What you can do is drop the soda, from the straw, onto his tongue. That way he doesn't have to strain those muscles anymore. His throat is getting weaker, and it's hard for him to suck through the straw. It's just part of the process, sometimes."

She opens up her bag, and says, "It's time for these, too. They're swabs you can soak in water, and then gently dab on his lips."

She checks his pulse and breathing, "Everything is normal. How do you feel, Richard?"

"I just want to go home, but these two donkey nuts refuse to leave."

His fingers are picking the blanket wildly.

"Oh Richard, you always make me laugh," Heather smiles.

I watch her finish cleaning up the tumor, grateful I didn't have to do it. She says, "Let's go sit down, and go over a few things."

We sit down; I hope she is giving us a timeframe.

Heather says, "His vitals are normal and he still is eating. I just don't know. He is so gradual. I have never seen anyone linger through the stages like this."

"Does he have to go through every stage the book says?" I ask, exasperated.

"No, I really thought after Tuesday, he would not be here today. Even the chaplain thought within a few days. I don't know what to say."

I'm distraught. "Well, what am I supposed to do? I have to go back."

"I'm sorry. I can't tell you when. Everyone is different, and he is much harder to predict than any other patient. We could be sitting here again next week. I don't know."

Mom interjects, "I can't believe how he is hanging on because that man was not a fighter. I know this is going to sound awful, but he was a big wimp."

Heather smiles, and then continues, "Due to the heavy picking, let's up his dosage a half a drop of each. It should relieve his anxiety."

She and Mom chat, but all I can do is think about the days to come and imagine how many there will be.

Heather leaves and Dad is asleep. Mom and I are tired and weak, so we sit, contemplating The Scene in front of us.

He starts to stir, and his voice gradually rises, "I'm hungry."

"You're hungry?" Mom says, surprised.

"Yeah."

The green numbers, 10:47, grin at me as I stride toward the fridge. I hit the microwave hard and say, "Fuck you! You can kiss my ass!"

*

"Come on, get this going. I have to get this started, and back to the shed."

"You've got to be kidding me?" I squawk back. "You are back on the mower?"

His hand begins to motion as though he is turning a key. "Come on, Molly, move me up so I can reach the pedal."

Mom has been in the laundry room for over two hours.

I open the door and ask, "What are you doing in here?"

"I'm ironing."

"For who, the whole neighborhood?"

*

He has been on the mower and in the truck all day,

these two recollections apparently his worst of eighty years.

His crackly voice becomes a moan, as he demands, "Ma, get my robe."

I walk to his side, "Dad, you don't have a robe."

With great certainty, he says, "Everyone has on white robes. I need my white robe. Please, Molly, go get my robe."

"Who is everyone?"

His hand reaches into the air, but no response.

"Who Dad? Who is there?"

"Skeeters, please take me into town. I have to get my hair done for the party."

"What party, Dad?"

"I don't know Skeets, but I have to get ready. Now, please take me into town."

"Dad, we are not going into town."

"Molls, I want to get my hair done."

I can't understand anything he is blubbering after that, but he is amused by whatever he is reaching for.

Dad always did look his best. His hair was perfect, and his wardrobe was color coordinated like no other man. Brown was his favorite shade, and in the winter he sported it well. In the summer he was much more vibrant, especially on the golf course. He had a shirt, pair of shorts, a hat, and socks to match, in every color. Now he wants to be dressed in white.

I come upstairs from a nice long shower and hear Mom say, "God dammit Dick, stop that."

His shirt is on the floor, and it looks like they are playing thumb war as their hands battle back and forth.

He slaps her arm hard and shouts out, "Fuck you, motherfucker."

Mom argues back, "You are a naughty man, very naughty."

I rush over, fed up with it all, and straight into Dad's face I scream, "That's it! I've had it! Now, you listen here, if you ever hit her again, you will be back in the nursing home before you know it. Do you understand me?"

He pretends to not comprehend. As always, he can't confront a mistake. This proves the reason he lies here, miserable, in defeat.

"We need a little joy in this house, and I need some fresh air. I'm going to go get Wrigley," I say with one foot out the door.

I explain the mood swings to Babe and Henry. I say, "The peace was overwhelming the last couple days, but today you would never know he went through any of it. And now, he wants a white robe."

Babe questions, "A white robe?"

"Yeah, he says he needs one because everyone is wearing them. I don't know."

Henry leaves, and then walks back into the room, "This will probably do."

He puts a plush white robe in my lap.

"Oh my God, you have a white robe," I say.

"Yeah, it has this little horse on the front, but you can tell him it's his chariot to Heaven."

Babe whispers, "Put it on him. See if it works."

This seems like too much of a coincidence, I almost don't like it.

With Wrigley in one hand and the robe in the other, I take short strides across the road. Zack and Lynn's car is in the driveway. I open the door and Lynn says, "Molly, I'm making you a plate, I went to the Chicken Dip."

Mom notices the cloth draped over my arm, and says, "They had a white robe?"

"Yeah. Can you believe it?"

My feet move me to the bed. Once I stand near him, I show him the robe, and say, "Dad, here is the robe."

He is picking away; not paying attention, but I say once more, "Dad, I have your white robe."

No response.

"Fine, but when you are ready for it, you let me know."

I march to the laundry room, shut the door, and put the robe on the hook. I look to the ceiling, "Unbelievable, we get the robe, and you still don't take him."

*

The back door opens, and though I am hoping it's someone cool, it turns out to be Claire. She always looks like she is just about to cry.

Mom says, "How are you Claire?"

She whines, "I'm all right."

Lynn, Mom, and I are playing cards, but it doesn't distract me from watching Claire sitting next to Dad.

Mom convinces her to eat some chicken, and says, "It's good, isn't it?"

Claire replies, "It's all right."

I focus back on the game, but before long, Claire comes over to the table and leans in, "I think we should take Dad to a cancer center."

"What?"

Childlike, she fires back, "I think they made a mistake. I think we should take him in and get a second opinion."

Lynn's mouth drops. Mom and I put all our attention on the game.

It's best to ignore such a remark.

Dad can hear her, but says nothing.

Claire continues, "I just don't want to think that we didn't do everything we could. That's my opinion."

Mom's eyes form slits, as she returns, "I did what he wanted. I brought him home. That *is* everything."

*

Once again, it's just him and me as night falls. He screeches, "Curtis, watch out! We are headed for the ditch!"

I interrupt his hallucination, "Dad, where are you?"

He yammers back, "The truck is in the ditch. It's raining. Curtis, Curtis! Hit the brakes. Stop! Please, Curtis."

My hand clings to his, "Dad, Curtis isn't here, but he is okay. Everything is okay. Go to sleep now."

"But Curtis is in the truck."

"Dad, Curtis is home, asleep. He is in bed like everyone else in the world, except us, we are still awake. Now please, close your eyes, and try to rest."

I'm weak, and his bag is getting heavier. The air is thick, as is the grass, and I'm tired. Through the trees and in deep bunkers, he keeps giving himself more shots than necessary to the pin.

Day 36

A bright white light shines in and opens my eyes. I'm on the couch. Unbelievably, he slept most of the night. There is a blanket of new snow outside. Today is the first day of spring.

I can see his hand reaching. I approach The Scene and see his bandage next to his shirt on the floor. I look to his hands, which are full of blood, and scream, "Oh no! Oh man! Oh shit!"

I run to the tumor to clean and cover it. Mom bellows from the hall, "What happened? What did he do?"

"Look at his hands. He was picking his tumor."

Mom grabs the baby wipes, and begins to clean him.

Blots of red blood on the white sheet take me back to a childhood canvas.

The warm breeze felt great on my skin, but it didn't last long. I was four when he said to me, 'Keep your feet out away from the wheels.' I was on the back of his bike, my arms tight around him, but my foot swung in, and the spokes caught it. There was no pain or sound. Dad was wearing a white-ribbed cotton tank top. All I remember is the fresh blood splatter on the pure white cloth, and then waking up to my mother's frantic cries in the hospital room.

Mom lifts up the sheet and yells, "Oh my! Oh, I'm going to get sick, Molly look."

Blood covers his thighs; it appears he picked at the catheter. It looks bad, I'm about to pull the catheter, when it hits me, I have no idea what I'm doing. I walk away and grab the phone.

Courtney says, "I need to come out and fix it. I will be there in forty-five minutes."

*

It's been an hour and a half and I say to Mom, "You realize Courtney is the one who will come, when, you know?"

Mom responds, "You mean, and she is taking this long?"

"That's exactly what I mean."

I sit in the chair and anxiety strikes. I can't sit here much longer.

"Mom, don't get mad at me, but I have to go to Little D's after this."

Mom hollers from the stove, "Oh no you don't. You are not leaving this house."

The doorbell rings an end to the morning.

Courtney tells me, "This happens sometimes. He is picking a lot. Take the sheets and tuck him in tight with his hands above. He will eventually get there if you don't watch him, but it'll slow him down quite a bit."

According to the hospice book, this picking occurs because he is agitated. This is common when the body is shutting down, due to the decrease in oxygen flow to the brain and metabolism changes. This restless task may indicate something is still unresolved or unfinished that is disturbing, and preventing him from letting go.

The signs of death are different with everyone. Some experience all the stages, others just a few, and others just the moment. There is a spectrum of experience.

Dad is hitting every stage with great detail. He always took a generous allotment of time for everything he did. If you commented about how long he was taking, he would purposely move slower. He loved to be a smart ass, especially when we were getting ready to go somewhere he didn't want to go. Mom and I would be in the car waiting. He would come out of the door and always go first to the fridge in the garage to get a can of pop. Next, he would approach the car, open the can, and take a nice, long, refreshing gulp. Finally, he would open the door, start to get in, and say, 'Oh, I forgot my…' He had many words at the end of the sentence – money, jacket, hat, keys. It was all a setup, just to postpone, if only for a few more seconds, entering a situation he had no hankering to be in.

Courtney says to Mom, "You have such a nice home, Tweedy."

Mom replies, "Oh my God, really, it is such a mess, you should see when I decorate for the holidays."

"Oh, I would like to see that. All right, he is all set. Call me if you need anything else."

She grabs her bag from the floor, "Okay Richard, keep those hands where they can see them. If the girls need me they will call."

She walks out the door, and I jump up, "Okay, I'm going to Little D's."

"Molly, you are not leaving this house," Mom screams.

I walk to the kitchen, "Mom, I can't take this anymore. My stomach is a wreck, I'm sorry but I have to go."

"God dammit, Molly, you are not my daughter. How did you end up like this?"

"Mother, what is wrong with you," my back falls against the counter, and I slide to the floor.

My head drops to my hands, "Fuck!"

Mom is crying, "Drugs, you do drugs? I did not raise you like this."

"Drugs?" I laugh. I can't catch my breath, but finally sigh, "Oh, Mom, please, open your eyes. My dad is dying right there in the goddam living room."

I rise up and point at The Scene, "Look, do you not see him? It's not like I'm shooting a needle in my arm. I need to calm down. Now I'm sorry, but I'm going."

*

I didn't stay at Little D's long; I felt bad about our fight. She hasn't spoken to me in the hour I have been home. My body is loose and my mind is fried. I pull the blanket up to my chin.

His arms and hands have lost a lot of strength. Clutching onto the rails, he pulls with all his might, but can't get himself up. He hollers, "Let's go home."

I do not reply to his need.

Within seconds he tries again, "Ma, Ma, let's go home. Come on, Ma."

Snow falls heavily outside.

"Come on Molly, please help your mom put me to bed,"

Mom commands, "Stop picking!"

"You get over here, and put me to bed. I want to go to bed, and I want to go now," he retorts.

Mom and I ignore him, until he finally fades off.

I am in the office, writing the words of his eulogy. I see the cars pull up, and then I hear Curtis.

"How's Pops doin' today?"

The rustling of their jackets is loud. My fingers are still quick on the keyboard. They are approaching Dad. Chloe's voice is much softer than her father's, "Hey Gramps', how are you feeling?"

Dad's voice is too crackled to understand and their voices become muddled as I concentrate, still typing.

I scroll up to the top of the page I have written and read it through. When I am finished, I notice that the house has become silent. I walk out to The Scene.

Mom has them interested in some movie on the television.

"Hey, there's Dee Dos," Curtis says.

I fall on the mattress, and study my notes of the past few days. I say to Curtis, "Get this, Dad said he saw a turd. He said it was a mile long."

Curtis laughs loudly, and with stretched out words, says, "Oh yeah, the turd story."

"There is a story?"

"Oh yeah. I remember it like it was yesterday. Grandpa Lucky was cleaning the bathroom and he walked out with a newspaper with a turd on it. It was curled up, but very long and hanging off the sides of the paper. Dad's remark when he saw it was, 'That turd has to be a mile long.' I can still hear the laughter echo through the bar."

"You were at The Avenue?" I ask.

Curtis continues, getting bigger and louder as he goes, "Yeah, it was hilarious. Grandpa Lucky said he had to show everyone because it was the most humongous piece of crap he'd ever seen. God, that was funny. I forgot about it."

Nate looks at Chloe, and says, "I told you, your family is fascinated by shit."

Mom responds, "Always been a Weasley trait. I never understood why everyone in this family is so interested in farts and poop."

The room fills with laughter that Dad can hear. I begin, "It's true. In fact one of my funniest memories of Dad is about a turd. It was Thanksgiving, and Mom sent Dad to the store to get something."

Mom jumps in, "It was brown sugar, and he got white sugar."

I reply, "Right, whatever. Anyway, when he got back from the store, he went outside to shovel the deck. It was cold out, and lots of snow. I was in the kitchen when Mom began to empty the grocery bags. She was not happy, and proceeded to the deck where she screamed at him for getting the wrong stuff."

Mom adds, "It was for my yams. It was supposed to be brown sugar."

Everyone laughs, as do I, but I finish, "There must have been at least three casserole dishes on the counter that Mom had just made. I will never forget when he walked in the door, and toward us. He was pissed. His face red from the cold, and he had on these thick brown gloves. He walked up to the counter, smashed his hand down, and little white and brown particles went everywhere. He yelled, 'Stick this in your goddamn yams.'"

I continue to explain, "It was a piece of dog shit. It was all frozen and he shattered it everywhere."

Everyone is laughing, except Mom.

She says, "Oh yeah, real funny. Man, that man was a piece of work."

Dad's voice is scratchy, as he shouts, "Curtis, I have to ask you something."

Curtis gets up and walks to him, "Yeah Dad, I'm here."

Dad explains, "Monday night there was a party."

Curtis replies, "A party? Was there cold beer?"

Dad says, "Ooh, cold beer."

He continues, "There was this little boy there. He was covered in grease. Do you know who he is?"

"I don't, Dad. Who do you think he is?"

"I don't know, that's why I asked you. Now, is the brake on? It's time to start the truck and go home."

His voice becomes softer by the second. I can't make out his whisper. I say, "What Dad? Say it again, Dad."

His mouth moves, but weakness has taken over most of his being, including his tongue.

"One more time, Grandpa," Chloe says.

He breathes out hard, "I want to go home."

Chloe replies, "You can go home, it's okay."

Cody, soon after, says, "Grandpa, it is okay, you can go."

We watch him in silence, intrigued by his motions. His eyes are so blue and glazed, "I promise, I will never ask you guys for anything, again, if you just take me home."

Curtis says, "Dad, if you are ready to go home, go ahead. It's all right Pops, you can go."

His gallery cheers him on, trying to boost his confidence. Encouraging him to finish this bitch of a course, and move on to broader, warmer fairways.

We all stand and say goodbye to each other, and then look at The Scene from the entryway. His hand is high in the air, his fingers frantically wiggling, as this moment becomes another timeless chapter. Curtis is the first to break the stillness. He opens the door and says, "We will be here earlier tomorrow, probably around two. See ya' later."

I follow him out, to feel the crisp air. Mom and I breathe it in for just a moment then return to The Scene. Mom exclaims, "Oh shit, Dick! How did you get that off so fast?"

"Are you kidding me? We just tucked him in!"

"Well, he managed to get out of it, Molly. I mean, look."

"God dammit, Dad. Why can't you just behave?"

I put on the green gloves, and begin to clean his tumor.

"Okay Mom, I'm done, you can put his shirt on if you want."

His arms fight her as she tries to cover his chest, "Richard, would you please let me put this on you."

His voice becomes strong, "I want to go home. I don't need it on to go home."

Mom yells, "You need it on so you don't pick."

His plea turns into a faint whisper, "I don't give a shit. Let's go home."

Day 37

Mom has been on the phone all morning. For some reason, everyone is curious about today's installment of the breakdown of a man. I guess they will have to be disappointed, because nothing is happening. His mouth is moving, but without words.

No one told me he was going to lose his voice. I knew he would get weaker and weaker, but I didn't realize he would become mute. His words were always simple but I never imagined they would disappear.

After a long shower and a short rest in solitude downstairs, I make my way back to The Scene. I find Mom fully reclined in her chair, head back, mouth open, and completely unaware of Dad's status.

Dad's shirt is on the floor with the sheet and the blanket, but luckily, his pillow is in his hands. If he didn't have the pillow, I'm scared to think what he would be holding, for he is completely naked with just a hose coming out of his penis. I quickly rebuild the bed.

It holds a soul, scoured, almost back to pure. Innocence at death must be as whole as innocence at birth. His skin is wrinkly, his body is scrunched up, even the catheter looks like an umbilical cord. He wants to leave this world the same way he entered it.

The door opens; Chloe and Nate walk in.

Chloe says, "We just came from my dad's house, and I have to warn you, Cody brought my mom."

I haven't seen Christy since I was about thirteen. She threatened many things upon my mother and our home. She was always a bit crazy. Mom told Curtis years ago, she didn't want Christy at the house, ever again.

Mom sees her first and says, "Oh, Christy is here."

She hasn't changed a bit—small, a dark complexion, and long, straight, black hair. Her face is more worn and rough than I remember. She smiles at me. She is wearing a pink sweat suit and trendy purple tinted glasses that don't quite hide the red of her bloodshot eyes. She is spaced out, obviously high on something.

"Molly Dee Dos, oh, it's so good to see you," Christy says, as she wraps her arms around me.

"Where's Curtis?" Mom asks.

"He didn't come," Chloe replies.

"What, why not? Is he coming later?" I ask.

"I don't think so. He said he had to do his taxes."

"His taxes?" Mom says. "He never mentioned that yesterday."

"I think yesterday was hard for him. I don't think he can handle it anymore," Chloe replies,

Christy says, "I think he will come back before the end. He is just having a hard day with it."

She languidly approaches The Scene, "Hi Richard. How are you, dear Richard?"

His hand moves forward and grabs the air. As

Christy's hand clenches his, she says, "Oh, he is already transitioning."

His head turns to her and his lips move, but no word forms. Chloe tilts her head and frowns, "So, he hasn't spoken since yesterday?"

"No, he hasn't."

"There is a whole bunch of food over here, if anyone is hungry," Mom yells from the kitchen.

Dad's eyes widen and he distinctly mouths the word 'hungry'.

"You want food, Grandpa?" Cody asks him.

His lips move, and he actually breathes the word, "Yeah."

Christy walks back to the bed with a plate with a drumstick on it, "Put him up more, and I will let him take a bite."

He eats the whole drumstick and motions for more. After four pieces of chicken, he takes his first spoonful of ice cream.

As Chloe feeds him, she notices her mom in the kitchen and whispers to me, "She isn't going to drink that, is she?"

I turn, to see Christy pouring wine into a glass, "Looks like it."

"I can't believe her, she can't drink," Chloe says furiously. "She is not supposed to drink. Why is she drinking that?"

Christy makes her way to the couch with a glass of wine and a plate. Chloe asks, "Are you going to drink that wine?"

"Oh Chloe, it's just a glass of cheap wine," Christy answers. "Give me a break."

I lie on the mattress and enjoy the familiar surroundings.

Mom hollers out, "So, you think Curtis will come back?"

"I don't know, Tweets. I can't believe he didn't come today," Chloe replies.

Cody says, "Yeah, especially when he got ready and everything. He took his normal two hours to get ready, and then he didn't even come."

"What? Two hours?" I ask.

Cody replies, "Oh, my dad takes forever to get ready. His hair has to be just perfect."

"Really? Curtis? He doesn't seem like that."

Chloe says, "Oh yeah, he even dyes his hair."

Mom yells out, "Your grandpa did too."

"Oh yeah, he did, I remember, I was real young. That's crazy. Curtis is just like his father," I reply.

Christy chimes in, "And it takes Curtis forever to decide what to wear."

Mom hollers, "Dick was like that too. I have to say, your grandpa cared a lot about the way he looked. He was a very snazzy dresser."

Chloe giggles, "Yeah, Grandpa's socks always matched his shorts."

I yell out, "Well, shit, he had over a hundred pair!"

Mom says, "A hundred? He had way more than that. I will never forget the time we went to Arizona to check out colleges for Molls. It was after we sold the condo and we stayed in a hotel room. We were gone for seven days; your Grandpa brought *twenty-four* pairs of socks, and only three pairs of underwear."

I laugh, "Oh my God, I was so mad at him. I will never forget being in the pool, and all the kids pointing up and laughing at Dad's tighty-whities hanging from the balcony."

Mom chuckles back, "Yeah, he washed them out in the bathroom sink and then hung them to dry outside. We were right above the pool, it was so embarrassing."

Everyone laughs, as I snuggle deep into my pillow. I'm almost asleep when I hear their voices again.

"I can have another glass of wine. I'm an adult. I'm your mother," Christy says.

Chloe yells back, "My mother? You were never my mother. An adult? You can't even go without it if you see a bottle. That's pathetic! Come on Nate, we're going home."

She grabs her coat and makes her way to The Scene, "Bye Gramps, I love you."

She kisses his cheek and darts to the door, "We're going home. I'll be back tomorrow."

Nate says, "I guess we are leaving. See you later."

He shuts the door behind him.

Christy sits down on the couch with her second glass of wine, as though she isn't getting up for a while. Cody submerges into his seat as well.

This is not good.

It's been a couple of hours, and Mom is still making a ruckus in the kitchen.

Dad's hand reaches high. Christy approaches him and says, "Richard, my dear, would you like something?"

No response, but his eyes are big and blue, as he

reaches for glory.

*

Finally, Christy and Cody are gone. I yell at Mom, "Man, I thought they would never leave."

"If they had stayed one minute longer I don't think I would have made it. I'm so done with all of this. I just don't understand why this can't end," Mom fusses.

I have no answer for her. She finally sits down. The television engrosses our minds and we drift off into fantasy.

Gabe walks in and points to the television, "Oh, I love this guy, he is so funny."

He approaches The Scene like the nights before, but once he sees how still Dad is, he joins us.

Mom finally says, "Oh my God, it's almost one. I need to go to sleep."

"Me too," I say.

I advance and softly kiss Dad's head.

Day 39

Mom and I have been weary. Neither one of us has moved much for almost two days.

"Molls, you have to do the tumor, I can smell it, bad."

"Okay, but you have to find some spray."

There is a very distinct smell. It has been lingering all day and seems to get worse by the minute. As I peel the bandage away, clumps of tissue crumble, and I realize its normally bubbly moisture is dried up and brittle. My fingers touch the inside of his chest like it's a routine I've known for years.

After a break downstairs, I am lying in Mom's chair. She hands me a bag of chips on her way into The Scene, where she straightens up the table of supplies. She says, "You are not going to like what I'm about to say, but I figured out what the smell is."

"Oh, yeah? What?"

She takes a great pause and then huffs and says, "It's death."

I analyze the scent for a moment.

"Like a funeral home," she describes.

I realize the deterioration of my father has seeped into the walls of our home. I reply, "Yeah. God, you are right. That's exactly what it is."

I see the shadows. Dark blotches cover certain spots. I can see death on the inside of the patio door. It is a fog, haunting and breathing the odor of expiration. Its presence is real. How long will it take to creep to its goal? Is this a demon taunting its prey? Where is the light that is supposed to shine eternally? Intrigued, I approach it, and wave my hands though its shade.

Mom asks, "What are you doing?"

"This is going to sound weird, but I can see it, too."

"See what?"

With a confident smirk, I reply, "Death. It's right here, just inside the door, lingering and waiting. The smell is even stronger here."

"I know, the smell is awful and it will only get worse. We have all these people coming over tomorrow. Are you sure you don't want to go out?"

"No, we need to be here. I'm not going anywhere," I say, as I grab the air freshener and try to kill the scent of my father becoming a corpse.

I should go work on the eulogy in the office but I don't want to leave Mom alone with it. There is a plant between the end of the patio door and the television, where it now stalks his being. My heart is beating fast. I challenge the lurking mass with my eyes. I can't look away from it.

His breath is labored.

It angers me to watch darkness drown our home and taunt his weakness.

*

The coldness of the sheets is inviting to my pathetic limbs. I curl up into a ball, while shivering turns to tears.

"I beg of you Lord, take him, please, take him. It's my birthday and all I ask is, you take him."

I whimper loudly, but shove the pillow over my mouth to hide the noise.

I'm calmed down, but still sleepless, tossing and turning recklessly, checking the clock every ten minutes.

It's 12:09 a.m., finally past midnight, but sleep is nowhere near. Thirty-three years ago, today, Dad saw me for the first time. Now I see him for the last. He began my life, and I am helping his end. A birthday is hard to play out when death oozes through the walls.

"Happy birthday, Molls," I whisper as my lids close, and I finally drift off.

Day 40

It's morning and I'm still here. My feet hit the hard wood floor, and I pound out to The Scene.

"Hi Dad."

"He didn't eat his breakfast," Mom calls from the stove.

"He didn't?"

"Well, he had a couple bites, but nothing like normal."

I study his motionless face. His eyes are closed.

"Okay, Dad, let's do your tumor now. We have a big day."

From the stove Mom bellows out, "Yeah, it's Molly's birthday. Happy birthday, Molls!"

She runs over and kisses me on the cheek. "Richard, do you know what today is?"

She grabs the brush from the table and combs his hair. He twitches, but the response is lifeless.

The tumor is extra red and puffy today. We may be getting through tissue and into his chest cavity. Deteriorated flesh, I clean every day; deeper, it becomes infectious with green and red bubbles disappearing by the second, as his body and soul both diminish before my eyes.

A process of death becomes a process of coming to life. The two are one, a transition from one spectrum to another. He exists in one, and he may exist in others. He travels through life and death, fighting for eternity. Time is a circle, not an infinite line. Dad is too concerned with the hours gone by – he is stuck in the ones past, and fearful of the ones to come.

*

I step out of the shower, and hear Uncle Mickey's voice.

"Hey Molls! Molls, are you down here?"

"Yeah, hold on."

I throw on my clothes and run out.

"Hey, happy birthday, kiddo. I thought you might like your birthday present now."

He hands me a baggie full of reefer.

"Sweet!" I say, as I hug him. "Oh my, God! Thanks so much."

"No problem. Lily and I are going to go up to the clubhouse to see if they will let us out on the course. We'll be back later, but I wanted to give you this."

"Oh yeah. I'm striking this up, right now. Thanks, Micks."

He runs up the stairs, and I go to my sanctuary for my ritual.

I hear the high-pitched voices as I pound up to The Scene. I am bombarded with hugs and 'Happy birthdays!'

Grandma says, "So, my sweetheart is thirty-seven today."

"Thirty-seven!" I scream.

Mom yells, "Mom, she is thirty-three, not thirty-seven."

The day goes by with people in and out, games, food, fun, and The Scene.

Chloe feeds him his third bowl of ice cream. His mouth is responding, but his eyes are still shut.

I approach his side and say, "Everyone is here. Like

always, there's a house full of people, and if it wasn't for you, Dad, I wouldn't be here. Thank you for bringing us all together. It's okay, you can go home now, Dad. Dad, I'm asking you for my birthday present. Please go home. I promise you everything will be all right."

He is not responsive to my plea.

I grab his hand and say with force, "Dad, squeeze my hand if you hear me."

His fingers are dry, cool, and paper thin, but squeezing my clammy palm tightly.

Day 41

The silver on the white pillow is again the first thing I see, as I make my way down the hall. Amy is already at the bed. She says, "Morning."

"Morning," I collapse into the chair. "So what's going on? How is he today?"

"I'm not sure, but he seems to be stronger than we think. He still has a lot of pee, too."

Amy goes on with an explanation, "A couple days before they go, sometimes, they will start to have a gargle in their throat. It's called a death rattle. That would be a sign he's close."

*

Amy is gone, and the room is silent, except for the distant water coming from Mom's shower.

Knowing he can't talk back, I feel more comfortable saying what I want to say. My hands grab the cold steel rail for support. I begin, "Dad, I want to thank you for the one thing you really gave me: my sense of humor. I want to write stories with it. Don't worry about Mom. She will probably move by me and I will make sure she is fine. I want to fall in love. True love; I know she exists and I'm asking you to help me find her. That's right Dad, *her*. I couldn't tell you sooner, you know how it is. And Dad, please, tell me what forty-seven means. That's it, Dad. Thanks. It's been incredible, just incredible; the best experience of my life. I love you Dad."

Not even a twitch for a response, but I know he heard me.

*

The smell of death is strong. Mom opens the windows, letting in cool air.

We sit in silence, Mom reads her book, Dad slowly dies, and I fade in and out of reality.

The Pastor's voice intrudes my nap. He says, "Thank you God, for blessing this family over these last few weeks, bringing us all together to fill Richard's last days here on Earth with much love; before begins his eternity with you. In Jesus name we pray, Amen."

*

Mom and I stare at the television, but I don't believe either one of us knows what we are looking at. I listen for the rattle.

Chloe opens the door, and enters The Scene.

"Hey, what's going on? How is he doing?"

"Not sure. No one seems to know anything," I answer.

"Well, Molly, they can't tell you when it's going to happen. They can't predict it," Mom snaps.

I reposition, sinking further into the cushion.

The door creeps open, and Curtis says, "Howdy? How's Pops doing?"

He walks to Dad's side, "Hey Pops, how you feeling?"

Dad does not respond.

"Hey Dad, it's me, Curtis. The date today is Thursday, March 25th. Tomorrow is Chloe's birthday."

Mom shouts out, "And yesterday was Molly's birthday."

Curtis repeats the line, "And yesterday was Dee Dos's birthday. Right now Chloe and Dee Dos and Tweets are all here."

Mom moves closer to The Scene, and I get up and walk to the foot of the bed. Curtis looks at me, then Chloe, and then back to Dad before he sighs, and says, "Dad, I been thinking about a lot of things these last few weeks. Memories from when I was a kid, working at The Avenue, and all the things we did. And, well, we had a pretty good life, Dad. And it's okay for you to go home. Don't be scared, and go in peace. We don't want you to suffer and hurt. We want you to go home, Dad."

He tries to clear his throat, holding back tears. His words tremble, as he continues, "I love you, Dad. You're the best Dad I ever had. So don't be afraid. Relax and when you are ready, Dad, go home."

I choke on my own spit, while trying to hold back emotion. I turn around, engulfed in the unbearable smell that has taken over the air. I stand in it for a moment to try to feel its energy, but then open the patio door. The air is cold and fresh.

"Oh, that feels so good," Chloe says, approaching the door, and breathing deeply.

We now stand in the kitchen and discuss Dad. My eyes only know one place to look. I watch him, but I don't understand the purpose of this watch, for I can't save him.

Dad twitches. I go to the bed, and see that his face is scrunched up, as though he is going to cry. His body is jerking rapidly.

"Oh my God! Someone help!"

Chloe and Curtis run over. Curtis grabs his body, "Dad, Dad!"

Dad calms down.

Curtis lays his hand over Dad's chest, "His heart is beating."

"God, I thought that was it," Chloe says.

"Me too, me too," I try to catch my breath.

Mom says to Curtis, "Do you know your sister's coming in tomorrow?"

"Katie?"

"Oh good, she needs to be here, now," Chloe says.

Mom asks Curtis, "Do you think maybe you could pick her up from the airport?"

"The airport?" Curtis laughs, "I don't know how to get there."

"You don't know where the airport is?" Mom snickers.

"No Tweets, I haven't been there since my honeymoon."

"Your honeymoon? Oh my God! Yeah, you would have no idea where you were going. You haven't been to the airport in over thirty years?"

"No, Tweets."

I interject, "Well, can you go with Mom to get Kate? I can't leave, and I don't want her driving there by herself."

"Oh Molly, I'll be fine," Mom rebuffs.

"Yeah, I can do that. What time you want to leave, Tweets?"

I need a break, so I slither away downstairs.

Fifty-five years old, lived in the same town all his life, and he doesn't know where the airport is. This place is driving me wacko. I don't know how I managed to grow up here. How can people live like this, with coloring books where all the colors are within the lines?

Back upstairs I lie, stretched out on the couch.

Mom nestles in her chair, and says, "Did you hear Curtis tell Dad that he was the best Dad he ever had? What a crock, I mean he's the only Dad he ever had."

I giggle, "I know, but you know what he meant, he was just trying to say goodbye."

Mom replies, "I can't believe he doesn't know how to get to the airport. What a dork."

"Yeah, now that's what I mean when I say *Midwest mentality*."

"Oh Molly, not all of us are like that."

"Oh no, not at all," I reply, sarcastically. "I'm just glad he can ride in with you."

"Oh Molly, I don't know why you don't think I can't drive there alone. I drove into the city for years when I worked."

"Mom, that was twenty-five years ago. Under the circumstances, I think it's best you don't go alone. Now drop it. I'm done."

She smarts back with something unintelligible, and searches for a television program to watch.

The patio door is still open, and clean air floats through the screen.

A noise persists from outside. It's coming from a light fixture that isn't turned on or even plugged in, but rattles constantly.

I feel teased. That's the sound Amy described, but it's not coming from him.

I watch the fixture, but it doesn't move; it just makes a sound. Everything around it is empty. The trees are bare, branches hanging lifeless in the air, and the grass is dry and brown. My exposed arm is getting cold, and the numbness creeps all the way to my nose as the night falls deeper upon us.

The rattle of the lamp is getting louder, faster, and more constant. I turn and look at Dad. He is breathing hard. The lamp rattle begins again. There is another sound in the distance, sounds like bells, drowning out the rattle, and getting closer.

It's wind chimes. Beautiful.

The rattle picks up again, closer, and persists.

Heaven is in the distance, waiting for death to deliver a new soul.

The chimes wax and wane, but the rattle is stable, it lingers, seeking its prey without pause.

Now Dad's breathing is heavy, it dominates for a moment, until the chimes start up, this time louder than ever.

Another noise comes in and I turn around to see Mom filing her nails.

She always had to do this in the middle of the goddam living room. Unbelievable! The worst sound ever.

My head is about to explode—the chimes, the file, the rattle, his breathing, the chimes, the file, the rattle, his breathing, the chimes, the file, the rattle, his breathing—I need to go downstairs.

*

I'm about asleep, when the door opens.

"Finally, Gabe is here."

Mom says, "No, it's Claire."

What an ending to a rough day.

"Hi, how is Dad?" she breathes with much effort.

She deliberately undoes the baby blue ties of her coat, and lays it over the chair, as though it is a difficult chore; she takes long strides to his side.

"Hi Dad, it's Claire. Can you hear me, Dad?"

Mom and I make eye contact to communicate our wonder, at how we came to be so fortunate, to deal with this at 9:30 p.m.

"How long has he been like this?" Claire asks as she repositions the chair next to the bed.

Mom replies, "Just the last couple days."

"What does the nurse say?"

"She really doesn't know when. But he has gotten much worse in the last few days," Mom explains.

"What are they going to do about it?"

"They are not going to do anything. It's part of the process."

"The process? Letting someone die is just a process? This is crazy, just crazy."

She rubs Dad's arm, "Oh Dad, I'm so sorry. I'm so sorry this had to happen to you. You don't deserve this at all."

I turn and look at Mom, who rolls her eyes.

Curtis's words are acceptance of Dad's new journey. Claire's words are complete denial. She pollutes this house with sorrow. Pure hearts understand: when it's time to go home, it's time to go home.

She sees all the papers on the couch, and asks, "What are those?"

"They are just notes for the eulogy," I reply.

"The eulogy! What eulogy?"

"Molly is going to give Dad's eulogy," Mom explains.

Claire, with her famous smirk, looks directly at me and says, "You are going to give it? Isn't it the pastor's job? I mean, what if you cry. Are you sure you want to take the chance. I mean, you don't want to have a breakdown and embarrass yourself, do you?"

I look right back at her, and say, "I'm not worried, I'll be fine."

The door opens, and Gabe walks through.

"Hello," he says, as he makes his way to The Scene.

Mom says, "Gabe, this is Dick's other daughter, Claire. Claire, this is Gabe, your dad's home care guy. Gabe has been great help with your dad."

Claire replies, "Helping him, what? Die?"

Gabe answers her, "I guess you could say that. Some people need help, like your dad."

She has no response as Gabe put his hands on Dad's arm. "Hi Mr. Richard, it's Gabe. Everything is real good. You seem to be doing fine."

He turns to me, and says, "Another few days."

Gabe walks to the couch and sits down. With Gabe

here, I can leave Mom for a moment and take a break, so I run downstairs to release myself from The Scene.

When I walk back in, I hear Mom's voice, "Oh, I hated that car."

Claire replies, "Why? I liked it."

"Oh God, the color was that awful baby blue."

I add, "And the seats inside were that color too, and they had that disgusting felt material. God, I hated that car. I remember the night he brought it home. I knew he was in big trouble, and he was. Mom was pissed."

"Why?" Claire asks. "He bought it with his money. It was his car, his choice."

Mom says, "That's why it looked the way it did. Cheap! If he bought it, he bought it because it was cheap."

Claire argues back, "There was nothing wrong with that car."

"Just like when we did the basement," Mom continues. "Everything down there, from the carpet to the shower, was the cheapest item in the store. We got in the biggest fights because he would find the cheapest tag, and that was the one we ended up with."

It is 11:30 p.m. Claire walks out of the bathroom, and says, "Tweets, the bathroom looks terrible. I'm surprised you let the walls look like that."

"Oh yeah, I know," Mom surrenders. "I haven't had the time to do anything."

Claire sits back down, and says, "It looks awful. So what are you going to do with it, Tweets? You aren't going to leave it, are you?"

"I'm sure I'll do something when this is all over."

"Yeah Mom, it's strange you left it this long. You're

normally a freak when it comes to that stuff," I say.

"Oh Molly, I am not."

"Everything Dad or I cleaned, you would redo. It made no sense for us to do anything. You are OCD."

"Oh Molls, I am not!"

Gabe chuckles.

Mom diverts, "You know, your dad had a good life. He always did what he wanted to do."

"Hey, what was the story, when he forgot you in Arizona?" Claire asks.

Mom recites, "We were in the van, and we stopped in New Mexico, at a gas station in the middle of nowhere. I went to the bathroom, and when I came out, the van was heading down the road."

I continue the story, "Yeah, I remember. Grandma was in the front seat with Dad. She said, 'Hey Tweedy' and Mom didn't respond. She repeated it a bunch of times, until I finally said, 'Mom isn't back here.' Grandma said, 'What?' so I told her again, 'Mom isn't back here.' Then Grandma starts yelling at Dad, and he turns the van around, real fast, and races back to the station. When we pulled up, Mom was sitting on the curb, waiting. Then we got down the road a little, and Dad had to pull over because there was a gigantic turtle in the road. He picked it up to carry it to the side, and it peed all over him!"

*

My hand glides through his hair as I kiss him, and say, "I love you Dad."

I turn to Gabe, and say, "Goodnight."

Claire's departing headlights shine through the front window as she backs out of the driveway.

What a quack.

Another emotional day done, my head hits the pillow and the cool sheets embrace me. The thought that he is going to die is a drum beating over and over, until finally, I get to sleep.

Day 42

The doorbell wakes me, and I hurry to The Scene. Heather is here checking him.

Like most days, I collapse into the chair, and once again ask the question, "So what do you think?"

"His vitals are good, and he still has a lot of pee," Heather replies.

Different day, same answer.

His eyes fight to open. Heather says, "Hi Richard. How are you today?"

"Thirsty," he mouths back.

"Water?"

"Pop," he mouths.

"I got it," I say, jumping up, and heading to the fridge.

I continue, "Wow, his eyes haven't been open in a day or so."

"They haven't?" Heather asks.

"No, he hasn't been awake."

"Kate is coming back in tonight," Mom says.

"Oh, that's great, that will really help," Heather replies.

I am relieved Kate will be here. I'm not sure how much more I can handle, without a breakdown of some sort.

As Heather gets ready to leave, I ask one more time, "So what do you think?"

"I really don't know," she replies. "He just keeps going. It's amazing he has lasted this long. I would think by Monday."

"I am glad Kate is coming," I reply.

"Yes, it is great she is coming back," Heather agrees, as she walks out. "She will be so glad she did."

"Call if you need anything," she says over her shoulder as she closes the door.

*

I had a nice hard shower and a fresh bowl of reefer; I'm ready to approach The Scene.

His eyes are open, so I say, "Would you like something?"

"Ice cream," he mouths.

I hear the front door open and I turn around to see Bridgett hunched over, struggling through the door with the baby.

She proceeds to the bed, "How's Gramps doing?"

"Not too good, but I don't know."

I head to the kitchen to prepare his ice cream.

I get halfway back to The Scene when Bridgett stops me, whispering, "I can't believe how bad he is."

"Yeah, I know," I say, as I approach the bed. "Here we go. I have your ice cream."

He opens his mouth, and I slide the spoon in. I get another scoop, he opens up, and I slide it in again. I begin to insert a third when I see the creamy substance in the back of his throat. I say to him, "Dad, you need to swallow your ice cream."

He doesn't respond to my concern.

"Shit, it's just sitting there," I yell out. "He can't swallow it."

"Well, we need to get it out of there," Bridgett says.

I grab the remote for the bed and bring the head of the bed all the way up. I grab the sponge swab to absorb the cream. I put the sponge past his tongue and into the throat. After a lot of dabs, I seem to have gotten it all.

"God, that was scary," I say.

Mom walks in, and asks, "What happened?"

Bridgett explains, and I take deep breaths. His mouth is moving around. He is trying to tell me he is thirsty. I get water in the straw, and put it against his lips. His lips shape the words, "More please. Thirsty."

"All right Dad, here we go."

I grab a swab, soak it in the water, put it on his lips, and he sucks it.

"Man, he is thirsty," Bridgett exclaims.

This next time, I soak the swab and let it dribble drops of water to his mouth. The moisture brings a glaze of peace into his eyes. I do this over and over, for about fifteen minutes, until he finally refuses the swab by nodding his head and pressing his lips tight together.

"You don't want anymore?"

He swats his hand angrily at me, and I say, "Okay, okay. I'm sorry, geez and crackers."

Bridgett approaches the bed and says, "Okay Gramps, we have to go."

His eyes look over to her and baby Hunter, but he doesn't have a response. He turns his head back and his eyelids drop.

"I love you, Gramps," Bridgett says, as she kisses his forehead. "Goodbye, Gramps."

She walks to the door, but turns back to memorize The Scene.

He can barely even swing the club. I'm doing everything I can, selecting his sticks, lining him up, and trying to get him closer to the green. He needs to finish this round.

The phone rings and I turn toward Mom. She grabs it and says, "Shit, it's Claire."

I grab the remote and turn the television down. Mom says, "Hello."

At first everything seems normal. Then Mom says, "What are you looking to do? Are you investing?"

That word caught my attention. Mom says into the phone, "Well, his name is Brad Kane."

"Why would you tell her that?" I ask loudly. I stand up, stretch, and walk to the kitchen. I open the fridge, grab the Coke, and chug about half the two-liter bottle, then make myself a sandwich.

Mom's voice rises, "Claire, what is the purpose of an IV if he is going to die anyway. If there was a chance he could live, then, yes, I would agree."

Mom pauses, and then says, "Claire, that's part of the process. They told us he would eventually not swallow. He is close. Why would you want to make him suffer any longer?"

I walk to the couch, sit down, and as I take my first bite, Mom yells into the phone, "I'm sorry, but I'm not doing it. I'm sorry Claire, this is the way it is. You have to deal with it."

A moment later she says, "Okay, bye."

She looks at me wide-eyed, "Geez and crackers, that girl is off her rocker. She wants me to call the nurse and get him an IV. Oh yeah, and at the beginning she wanted to know about my financial guy, and then she said Dad may want to tell us something, and an IV could make him talk again. Oh my God, I am so mad. I have to call Shells."

She dials the number and repeats the whole conversation to Shelly.

I text Kate the details of what was said, and get a response:

She's up to something.

*

It's 5:03 p.m. I'm watching Mom run around, cleaning. The poor sink has gotten the worst of it. I have the hospice book open on the coffee table. Every time she walks by, she closes it. I open it back up, and when she zooms by, she closes it. The counter has been reorganized five times in the last half hour. She is now outside cleaning the windows.

She is driving me crazy. I'm going to lose it. She needs to stop.

I say, "You need to calm down and take a break. You are out of breath."

"Oh, Molls, I'm fine, I need to do something. I can't just sit around," she says, still wiping and huffing.

"Whatever. You should think about your heart, and how careful you should be, especially with your husband practically dead in the living room."

I get up and head to the stairs.

Soon, Mom calls down to me, "They're actually here on time!"

When I emerge, Curtis greets me, "Food. I got food."

He turns to the living room and I see Christy behind him, still wearing her pink sweat suit and purple tinted glasses.

In a soft, far away voice, she says, "Hi."

We are all eating when the front door opens again. It's Claire. Not one of us pauses to greet her; we continue chomping our food. She makes a plate and sits down, away from us.

"Well, we need to get going soon," Mom says.

Oh God, I am going to be alone with Claire and Christy.

I find my phone and text Chloe:

Where are you

Before I know it, Mom and Curtis are gone.

"Molly, he feels really warm," Christy says, standing at the bed.

His fingers are picking badly at the blanket. I touch the back of my hand to his head, and his sweat dampens my skin. I say, "Yeah, he is very warm, and picking too much."

Christy walks away and Claire moves in and says, "What do you mean?"

"Well, he seems upset and when he gets upset, it's bad."

"What does that mean?" she hollers back at me.

"Here are some cold towels to cool him off," Christy says, as she hands me a couple.

Claire, not wanting to participate, turns to her food and says, "I don't understand any of this."

His arms are moving rapidly, his fingers going crazy, picking and grabbing everything. Christy and I are trying to control him; Claire watches from afar.

"Okay, let me give him his drops," I hurry to the kitchen to get them ready.

"What are those for?" Claire asks.

"They will help calm him down."

"Calm him down? I don't see what he is doing is so out of the ordinary."

"Well, the way he is picking means he is agitated, and if he gets worse, it could be bad. These drops will help."

I put the drops against his gums. I rub his cheek, hoping they sink in and put him to sleep.

Christy, still cooling him off, says, "His whole body is hot. I think he has a fever."

"Okay, I will call hospice."

I run to the phone and dial.

"Angel Hospice, this is Courtney."

"Hey, Courtney, it's Molly, calling for my dad. He is very hot and seems to have a fever. He is picking like crazy and is very upset."

Claire rolls her eyes, "Upset? He's not upset."

I hang up the phone, and run to the fridge to get the drops. Claire asks, "Now what are you doing?"

"She told me to give him more drops, to calm him

down."

"More drops? Why more?"

"What I gave him was just the minimum. He needs more to calm him, and if this doesn't work, she may have to come out."

"Come out for what? I don't see what is so bad."

I walk over to The Scene. Christy is trying to hold him back. His arms are fighting and winning over her strength. I open his mouth, and place the drop on his gum. I say, "Okay Dad, relax. Just relax. Let this help you sleep."

Claire says, "I can't believe I'm watching this. Is this really happening? Poisoning my father before my very eyes, and I'm watching this."

She keeps going, but I don't hear any more, until her final cry gets my attention, "This is crazy. I can't be a part of this."

Still rubbing his cheek after the final drop, I focus on Christy, who is helping. She brings fresh towels. She gently wipes his face and arms. He grabs her arm while his lips move up and down frantically, but no sound comes out.

"Shit, he has never been this bad," I say.

"What do you mean *this bad*? He is doing nothing wrong," Claire announces.

Before I can scream, Christy grabs my arm, and says, "You are doing great. You know what is going on with him, don't let her bother you."

I reply, "Okay, let's try a sponge. Maybe I can get him to focus, while the drops sink in."

I get a swab and soak it with water, before dabbing it on his lips.

I say to him, "Come on Dad, open your mouth, you need to drink."

His mouth opens, and I gently press the swab on his tongue, so a few drops seep out. My hand springs back as my heart races with worry. *What if those few drops are too much?*

"Dad, can you move your tongue around? You have some water on it."

He helps the small amount of liquid disappear, easing my mind for a moment.

Christy says, "There you go. Feeling better. He feels cooler."

"But his hands are still moving. That's a bad sign."

"Yeah, I know," Christy answers. "He is really upset and the more he grabs the more upset he gets."

"Shit, those drops should have stopped it, but it's getting worse."

His body starts to move around angrily, and he grabs for Christy.

Claire walks over and says, "What's he doing?"

"He is upset and it's getting worse," I say, while trying to pry his hand off Christy's arm. "This is why I needed to give him the drops sooner. The longer you wait, the worse it becomes. Dammit, come on Dad, let go."

I finally unclench his fingers from Christy's feeble limb.

"Fuck me," I say under my breath as I race to the phone.

"Hi Courtney, it's Molly again."

"Hey Molly, what's going on?"

"He has gotten worse. He is grabbing with a lot of

strength and trying to get out of the bed."

"Okay, let's give him another dose, like before, and if it doesn't work, you will have to use a suppository."

"A suppository? We have those?"

"Yeah, it should be in the kit with the drops."

I walk back to the fridge, open the box, and see them at the bottom.

Claire yells, "A suppository, no way!"

I try to listen to Courtney's directions over the phone, but Claire's words are muddling the message, disrupting my mind. I get the drops ready, and Claire begins again, "More? You've got to be kidding me, right?"

I ignore Claire, as I pass her and run to the bed. I press the dropper into his gum. In my one ear, Courtney is going on about how to use a suppository. In my other ear, Claire has really got me rattled with her chanting, pleading, and crying.

"Why does he need so many of those? That is absurd. What is it called?" she hollers at me.

I don't say anything, but give her a look, as though she should shut her mouth. I turn around and walk back to the kitchen.

The phone is still to my ear, as Courtney asks, "You got it all?"

Having not heard one word, I answer, "Got it. I will call you if I need to."

Chloe comes through the front door, "I'm so sorry, I'm late."

"Oh my God, where have you been? I have to go downstairs, please check on him."

I sprint down for a quick breath of sanity. I look in the mirror and scream, “How in the *fuck* did I get myself into this one? This is just plain stupid. Stupid!”

I continue to shout, puffing away my madness.

I take a deep breath before I head back up to The Scene.

“Where’s Claire?” I say as I walk to the bed.

“I’m leaving,” she snipes. She is standing by the door, putting on her coat.

“You’re leaving? You’re not going to wait 'till Kate gets here?”

She shakes her head and then wraps it with her scarf.

“No,” she says, and walks out.

“Wow! She has got problems,” I shout.

I start to tell Chloe about what Claire had been saying, but then I notice that Dad is calmed down. He is asleep.

“Yeah,” Christy says, nodding at Dad. “He settled down, and dosed off.”

“Sweet, finally, he will be out for the night,” I reply.

Chloe jumps in, “Now what happened? What did she say?”

I hear the creak of the back door. “Hello,” Mom hollers. “We’re home.”

Chloe runs over to hug Kate, “I’m so glad you’re back.”

Curtis walks over to the bed. His hands come out of his pockets. He sets one on the rail and the other extends out to Dad’s shoulder, “How’s Pops doin’?”

“Where’s Claire?” Mom asks.

“She left,” I reply.

"She left?"

"Yeah, she has got major problems."

"You are just realizing this now?" Kate laughs.

"I didn't realize what a bitch she is."

In a mocking tone, Kate whines, "Her Daddy is dying and no one can fix it."

Curtis hollers, "Come on, come on, this is hard on her."

"Molls, what do you mean, she has got problems?" Mom asks.

I explain what happened while they were gone.

Kate ventures to the bed, "Hi Dad."

His breathing is hard and his eyes are closed. She kisses his forehead and strokes his hair.

She says, "I have told you guys over and over, Claire is bad news. When her true self comes out she is just plain vicious."

The room is silent; we concentrate on Dad's breathing.

Kate says, "He is so much worse. He is close."

"We have thought that for days," Mom replies.

"Days? More like weeks," I comment.

"Molly, did you do the tumor tonight?" Mom asks.

"No, not yet."

"That smell is bad, you need to do it."

"All right," I turn around and begin my preparation with some gloves.

It is plain, brown and dry, not bubbly and green like before. All the juice is gone. Everything making it unique and fearful has disappeared.

Day 43

Footsteps awaken me, so I grab the blanket and bury myself in the couch.

"I'll be back later," I hear Mom say as the back door shuts.

"Where is she going?" I ask Kate, as I rise.

"To the store. She said she had to refill her prescriptions."

The phone rings. "Shit. Who the hell is that already?" I say.

I don't recognize the number, so I don't answer, but I listen to the message. With a lifeless voice Claire says, "Hi, it's me. I need someone to call me back immediately. I did some research and found out that the Haldol drug is why Dad can't swallow."

I shriek, "Oh my God, what is she talking about?"

I dial her back. I say to Kate, "What a fucking nightmare she has become."

Claire answers. "Hi Claire, it's Molly. What's going on?"

"Well, I have some bad news," she replies. "I looked up Haldol on-line and found out its number one side effect is difficulty swallowing. You need to call the nurse and change it, and see if we can get him an IV, so he can talk."

"Claire, he is dying," I explain. "The nurse told us he would eventually not be able to swallow. It's part of the process. This is it. Why can't you understand? Do you want to prolong his agony?"

Kate walks by and pumps her fist—*one for the home team.*

"You want me to understand that my dad is dying?" Claire starts in. "Why would I want to do that? I want to help him. What if he needs to tell us something? Now he can't, but if we get him an IV then maybe he can talk again."

"Why does he need to talk, when he is dying? He can't be saved."

"But Molly, that drug is killing him. You are killing him. I mean this is as close to assisted suicide as you can get. I can't believe you are killing our father."

I look at Kate, and say, "Hey, according to Claire, this is an assisted suicide."

Kate yells, "What? That woman is crazy."

"I'm not killing him, I'm helping him die," I reply to Claire's remark. "It's not what I want to do, but I have no choice, and at least I'm here with him, doing it."

"Yeah, that's exactly what you want to do, help him die," she rebukes me. "So you admit it?"

"Claire please, I'm not going to have this conversation with you because I need to tend to our dying father now."

"I just want to say one last thing, to help you realize what's right. If you don't stop this, you will regret it for the rest of your life. You are killing him. Don't you understand? You can change this whole situation. Call the nurse and get him an IV. Even better, let's just take him to the hospital."

I laugh.

"What's so funny? What did Kate say? What did she say?"

I'm boiling as I make my last remark, "She said nothing. I was laughing at your stupid comment. I'm done with this conversation. I am doing what Dad wanted. He wanted to come home, and die here in his house, and I'm not going to do anything to change it. Goodbye."

I hang up the phone. Kate says, "What a bitch."

"Man, you were right about her. Shit, now what do we do?"

Kate shakes her head with a smirk, "We do nothing. Screw her."

Where the hell does she get the right to show up for the last few holes? She hasn't been within the ropes. She has barely made it to the gallery on most holes, and now she thinks she can call the shots. She wants him to quit, but I won't allow it. Challenging conditions hold up his game, but it doesn't mean he forfeits. As his caddie, I will lead him to victory. As his daughter, I will guide him home.

A joint is calling, so I say to Kate, "Would you like to join me downstairs? "

"After that, I can't think of anything better," she says, and follows me. "I can't believe she is acting like this. She is getting out of hand."

*

The ritual is finished. We walk by the bar on the way to the stairs. Kate says, "Let's check out the booze."

We pull bottles out and make our way up with fists full of alcohol. Kate reaches the kitchen counter and makes herself a drink.

It's 3:00 p.m., when we hear the back door open and Mom walks in.

"Where have you been?" I ask.

"Molly, I had a lot of things to do." She goes straight to the fridge, "You girls want a sandwich?"

Kate yells, "Tweets, you need to sit down and relax. Plus, we need to tell you what happened while you were gone."

Mom notices the liquor, and says, "Oh man, you guys are drinking. Now what?"

"Just come over here and sit down, Tweets. Claire called, and Molly had to deal with her craziness. Molly did a great job handling her. Claire thinks we are assisting suicide. She thinks we are killing Dad."

"What exactly did you say to her, Molly?" Mom inquires.

Kate interjects, "Tweets, she wants him to be able to talk for some reason."

"You think she is up to something?" Mom asks.

"Oh Tweets, don't be so naive," Kate replies. "Of course, she is up to something."

*

Back up the stairs from a small break, I notice a familiar light blue object on the counter. I scream, "What the hell is that? Why is it there?"

"What?" Kate asks.

"That hair dryer. I have thrown it out twice because it

spits out fire, but Mom, for some reason, wants to keep it."

From the hall Mom shouts, "It doesn't need to be thrown away. I can put it in the garage sale."

"Mom, it is broke. You can't sell it."

Kate smiles, shaking her head, "Yeah Tweets, that's crazy, throw it away."

"I am!" I shout, as I grab it and rush out the door into the garage. My arm flies up as I chuck it into the trash bin, and yell, "I'm so done with you and your stupid, fucking, baby powder blue, bullshit!"

*

Night falls. His breathing is heavy. I peel off the tumor-juice soaked bandage from his chalky, crumpled skin.

"Man, it's really draining, so different from last night," Kate says. She takes the stained shirt out the back door and into the garage.

I soak up the fluid with balls of gauze, the size of small plums, then carefully dab the inner core. It's a tunnel, becoming deeper and closer toward the end of its path.

Kate, back at my side, hands me tape to seal the opening on the side of his chest. I say, "Look, his nipple is almost gone. I remember when it barely touched it."

Mom comes up, and says to Kate, "I think we should sleep out here now because I don't want her alone when it happens."

Mom is on the air mattress, and Kate and I each take a couch. His breathing keeps me up most of the night. Mom and Kate toss and turn as much as I do.

Day 44

A harsh gargle wakes me.

This is the death rattle.

I spring up to his side. Kate says, "What is that sound?"

"I don't know. He seems to be okay. His breathing is still heavy."

Kate says, "Okay, I have to go to the bathroom."

His eyes are shut, but his mouth moves.

I say, "Dad, can you hear me?"

His lips, the only thing responding, show me he is thirsty. I wet a sponge swab, and press it to his lips. His mouth opens, and I carefully wet the inside. As I bring the swab out, it is covered with white flakes.

"Gross, what is that? Disgusting!" I scream.

I look in his mouth and see a huge scab of skin on the back of his throat.

I whisper to myself, "Oh my God, this can't be good. You could choke on that."

"Shit! Kate, we have problems," I shout.

"Okay, I'm brushing my teeth."

She walks out with a toothbrush in her mouth.

"Look inside his mouth."

She bends down and looks, "Yuck! What is that?"

"I don't know."

"Get the flashlight."

"Oh, good idea," I say, grabbing it from the table.

Kate says, "Wow, it's huge. It's like a big, old scab."

"I know, and it's flaking everywhere. I'm calling hospice."

Courtney tells me to, cautiously, use a swab and take out the scab. I slam the phone in the couch, and yell, "Fuck me! I'm so tired of all this. We have to get it out of there."

"How are we going to do that?" Kate sounds baffled.

"Hell if I know. Courtney says, with a swab."

Mom shouts from the hallway, "What is going on out there?"

"Come here and look at this."

I point the flashlight in his mouth, and say, "We have to get *that* out of there."

Mom says, "Gross. What is it?"

"It's a scab I have to peel off and pull out. Shit! I don't see how this is possible."

Mom turns and walks into the kitchen, asking, "What do you girls want for breakfast."

"You still have those bagels?" Kate asks.

"Yeah, we have a lot."

"What about that strawberry cream cheese?" I yell.

"Yeah, we got it."

Kate and I run to the kitchen and make bagels.

I devour mine while thinking of the best way to get the scab out.

We are back at the bed. Kate holds the flashlight, as I use a swab to probe at the back of his throat. Flakes fall, but there are layers and layers of hard scab, and then layers of flaky scab. I get nothing but flakes for thirty minutes. A small chunk finally falls, and I scream out, "Shit, it fell on his tongue."

My hand shakes desperately. Kate gasps, "A tweezers. Tweets, where are your tweezers? Oh, wait a minute, I have some."

She darts down the hall. She returns and hands them to me.

"Shit, this is not working. I can't get it."

"Just keep trying," Kate says.

He coughs, and the chunk moves toward his throat.

I jump up and say, "Shit, he is choking."

"No he's not," Kate yells. "Not yet, but this is scary, and you are freaking out. Look, the chunk is right there."

With one more try, I remove it, and say, "I'm done. I'm calling Courtney back."

"I'm done too," Kate breathes deeply.

Mom, still in the kitchen, yells, "Yeah, me too. I'm done."

Kate and I stare at the television while we wait for Courtney to come.

I'm just praying time goes by fast enough for her to get here before he chokes on that thing.

About two hours later, Courtney rushes through the door, "I'm so sorry. I had another call before you. It took longer than I expected."

"I'm just glad you're here, and he hasn't choked on it. Please, get it out of there," I plead.

"Wow! That is huge," she says, as she puts the swab in his mouth.

She skillfully uses her fingers to pull out a pear-shaped scab, the size of the back of my hand. It's gray and green on the bottom, with brownish red clumps layered to the top, where a pile of dead flakes nestle.

Kate says, "It's bigger than it looked."

Courtney replies, "Yeah. I think that's the biggest one I've ever seen. Wow! I can't believe that. This poor guy has had some issues."

Mom chuckles from the stove, "Oh, I believe it. That man has more problems."

Courtney continues, "These scabs happen so fast. You really want to check his mouth, and wet it with a swab constantly. I'm going to check his vitals and his heart to see what's going on."

"He has been out since Friday," I tell her. "Does that mean anything?"

"He is getting closer. His vitals are still good. His breathing is fluctuating a little, but with him, it's hard to say. I'm thinking within the week."

Mom has been running around fussing this whole time. She sees the bedside wastebasket out of its place. She approaches it, notices the scab, and says, "Was that the thing in his throat?"

Courtney replies, "Yep, it sure was."

Mom responds, "My God. That's horrible. Boy, it's just one thing after another, isn't it Richard?"

*

The day goes on with movies and naps, as we lie with Dad and watch his features become more defined.

The door opens and Christy walks in, "Hi, all. How we doin' today? How's my dear Richard?"

She approaches The Scene without hesitation. Curtis walks in, "Howdy everyone, how's Pops today? Hi Pops. It's me Curtis."

"He hasn't been awake since Friday," I say.

Christy, in her sweat suit and the same purple glasses, replies, "Really? He is very close."

"You think so?" I ask.

Her hand touches his shoulder as her head tilts at me, "Yes. He won't wake up."

"I know, but he could lie like this for weeks."

She smiles as she debates my worry, "No he won't. His time is here."

Cody walks through the door with a puppy, and asks, "Can I bring him in?"

"Yeah, that's fine, but don't let him mess anywhere," Mom tells him.

"Just hold him, Cody," Curtis says. "Don't let him down."

He hands me the pup, and says, "Here, hold him while I go see Grandpa."

Curious, the little one stands on my lap, sniffing the air

around. I can feel his heartbeat. It's such a lively thump, excited to explore, play, and live. He lies down, and spreads his front paws out, off my knees. His head falls on his paws as he huffs a puppy breath. My fingers glide through the pup's hair.

"Have you talked to Claire?" Kate asks Curtis.

"Yeah, she called me yesterday," Curtis says, hesitant, "I think she just doesn't know how to handle this. It's a lot for her."

"It's a lot for all of us," Kate replies. "She's not the only one. Where has she been anyway? I'm here. You're here. Molly's been here over a month. Where is she?"

"It's Claire, everything is twice as hard for her," Curtis shrugs.

"That's bullshit," Mom says. "Deal with it, already."

I massage the pup's neck and investigate his little features.

After about an hour of discussing Claire, Dad, and all the bullshit, Curtis gets up and puts on his coat. He approaches Dad, and says, "Dad, I'm gonna' go now. So if you are ready to go home, go ahead. If you are not ready yet, I will see you at the end of the week. I love you, Dad."

Christy doesn't seem to be moving, but Curtis is already at the door. Curtis says, "Come on, let's go."

"I'm staying the night and helping the girls, remember?" Christy responds.

My head pops up.

What the fuck is going on now? This can't be. This just can't be.

Cody tries to take the pup from my lap, but I stop him and whisper, "Take her home. She cannot spend the night.

Please, Cody."

I finally hand over the dog.

Cody walks to the door, saying, "Come on Mom, let's go."

She sighs, "I'm staying here, Cody, I told you that when we left. Go get my bag."

I turn to Kate and whisper, "Fuck, she has a bag."

Mom yells from the kitchen, "Christy, go home, we will be fine. All he does is sleep. Really, it's okay."

She moans back, "But I thought we could have a girls' night."

"We will probably be asleep within an hour," Mom responds. "Curtis, you guys go home."

Curtis says, "Come on, Christy."

She gets up, and says, "Yeah, I'm tired too."

As soon as the door shuts, I yell out, "Holy shit. I can't believe she was going to stay the night. Could you imagine?"

"No. I can't," Kate says, relieved.

Mom sits down and reclines her chair as she says, "What a dork, like I'm going to let her spend the night in my house."

Kate and I curl up in our chairs, giggling. Within seconds we are all asleep, but within minutes the phone rings.

Mom gets up to answer it. Soon she replies, "I am sitting down. What is it, Shells?"

I look at Kate with a shear of the eyebrow.

What the fuck is it now?

Kate and I stare at her, while she listens to the phone closely. "You got to be kidding me? Oh my God. When was this?" Mom shouts as she ejects from her seat, and slaps her thigh. "Jesus Christ, that asshole! What an asshole! That's why she wants him awake; to sign it over, probably."

She turns to Kate and me.

"Mom, what happened?" I ask.

"Your dad told Shells he paid off the mortgage on Claire's house."

"What?" Kate screams. "He did what?"

She gets up, and starts toward the kitchen. "He did what? Ask her when," she continues, pouring herself a drink.

Mom doesn't reply, for she is too involved in the words she is getting from Shelly. Kate walks back out, and looks at me, "How did he do that? I can't believe he would do it, but it does explain how she lived for so long without a job. If she had no house payment, it makes sense. She is losing her lifeline. He probably fed her money her whole life."

As Kate rambles on, I lose track of the both of them as my eyes study him. His face is white, the skin is clenched in, stuck on his cheekbones. It resembles an alien's face, with tight skin and an oval shaped head.

The shape of his core is something we can't interpret. If he can hear the conversation at hand, he knows this is the last lie. Is this his biggest secret? He was cheap his whole life, never gave. He always did what he felt like doing; never thinking about the feelings of others – except for one, it seems.

I was the last thing he ever wanted. I disrupted his life and Claire's. To make up for it, he took care of her. What did I get? A hospital bed with an alien form that is afraid to die, for he assumes hell is his future.

I get up and approach the bed, "Oh Dad, what did you do?"

His breathing is hard. I see his throat moving up and down. His neck is thin. All I see are the bones sticking through his almost gray skin.

Kate shouts from the counter, "Oh my God, where are all the pills?

I turn around, "What?"

Kate is waving Dad's pill basket.

"This thing is like, half empty," she says.

I can tell from where I am that there are bottles missing. They used to rise above the basket, and now I don't see any.

We are silent for a moment then Kate shouts, "Christy!"

"Oh my God, it was!" I reply

We can't help but laugh. Mom throws the phone hard onto the couch and walks to the bed.

"Well, Richard, I always knew you were a piece of work, but I never would have thought. The way you are with money, and you paid off her mortgage. My God! What the hell else did you do?"

"He can't answer you," Kate replies. "And even if he could, he would divert it anyway. You know how he is. Now, what exactly did Shelly say?"

Mom replies, "She said that about ten years ago or so, he stopped by and was distraught because he had just paid off Claire's mortgage. He told them, 'If my bride found out about this she would kill me. Please don't tell my bride, but I have to get it off my chest.' Shells said they promised him they would never tell me, but now she felt I should know because of the way Claire is acting."

"How could he pay off her mortgage?" Kate asks, exasperated. "That's a lot of money. You would have known."

"I don't know. Our finances were completely separate, but you know Dad, I'm sure he exaggerated the truth. He always did when it came to money."

Kate agrees, "Yeah, I'm sure it wasn't too extravagant, but he obviously did something, and if he did, there has to be some kind of proof."

Mom replies, "There's a whole bunch of brown paper bags in the storage area, in the basement with his receipts and bank statements."

Kate runs to the stairs. I follow, saying, "Wait for me."

Mom says, "Oh Dick, I can't believe you would do that."

We sprint down the stairs, as Kate yells, "I'm going to kill him if he did."

"Well, at least then he would finally be dead," I reply.

We chuckle, as we enter the storage room. Kate points and says, "Here they all are."

I reply, "Oh my God, all those bags?"

We make our way back up the stairs, with our arms loaded. I can hear Mom on the phone again.

She says, "I know, Judy. I know. Can you imagine what else I may not know about? What he could have done? Oh, Richard, you've got me so pissed right now."

I drop four bags filled with papers, and say, "I hope we find something, and if we do, I'm glad he is right here to see it."

Kate laughs, "Yeah Dad, you hear that?"

"Good thing your hearing is still good. I mean, you can't see, or talk. You never talked. The only thing you ever did was pay off Claire's mortgage," I announce.

Kate dumps a bag out and papers fly everywhere. We begin to look for clues of a big withdrawal he may have made. We sort the bank statements from the receipts, and the paycheck stubs, and all the other nonsense we find. It has been a couple hours, but there is nothing too interesting. Mom, Kate, and I are delirious as we make jokes about the situation. We're laughing hysterically when the front door handle jiggles. I see blondish hair through the glass, "Oh shit, it's Claire."

Kate jumps up and darts toward The Scene. Mom yells out, "You've got to be kidding me."

As the door opens, we realize it is actually Leslie. Once inside, she asks, "What's so funny? I heard you laughing from the driveway?"

I say, "Oh thank God, it's you. I thought you were her."

Mom, Kate, and I start laughing and can't stop.

Leslie checks his blood pressure, as she asks for the fourth time, "What happened?"

Kate and I are rolling on the floor, holding our stomachs, while Mom attempts to talk.

Leslie says, "His blood pressure is very low. He really doesn't look very good either."

I reply, "Well, he has had a rough day."

Mom cackles again and tears fill her eyes. Kate says, "All right, all right, tell Leslie what we found out."

Leslie's facial expression tells me she doesn't find the news as important or as amusing as we do. She says, "You are so sleep deprived, this whole thing has you guys nuts."

Kate replies, "My dad was an asshole his whole life and now we find out he wasn't like that to everyone."

Leslie looks serious, "You know, he can hear everything you guys are saying."

Kate yells out, "I don't care. He needs to hear this. He had it so easy."

"He sure did, up until the very end, too," Mom responds.

Leslie says, "I'm sure he is sorry."

I laugh, "A little late now."

Leslie states, "This is what happens when someone dies, especially in this detail and length. You were bound to find out something. Just be glad this is all it is."

Mom sighs, "Oh my God, Richard, if there is more. I'm telling you, I can't believe any of this is happening. I'm done. I'm just done."

I say, "Me too, this is getting worse. This whole Claire thing is bad. She says I'm committing assisted suicide by giving him those drops. Friday night, I gave him, like, four in a row, and she saw it."

Leslie replies, "All three of you are acting crazy. You have been cooped up in this house, surrounded by his death, and it's finally gone to your head. Don't let Claire bother you. Just let her be. Let her think what she wants. Ignore her. Don't answer her."

Changing the subject, I say, "You know what happened earlier? We had to call the nurse out."

Leslie asks, "What happened?"

I tell her about the scab. She says, "Sounds like you guys have had an interesting day. What you really need is sleep. I'm going to leave, and let you guys get some."

Walking out the door, she says, "Take some pictures of his tumor. Just to have, in case Claire really is crazy."

"That's a good idea," Kate says.

We start right in, turn off and on different lights, and capture the tumor from all angles. A small lamp makes the room very dark, but captures the colors perfectly. After the shoot I go through, the now robotic, detailed process of cleaning and wrapping it back up.

"This is what we get, guys," I announce. "Now, we stand here and clean his tumor. This tumor is guilt. That's what it is, it's not cancer, it's guilt."

I finish bandaging.

"You're right, Molly," Kate says. "That's why he's still lying here."

Mom replies, "Well, he can lie there all he wants, that's what he deserves."

I yell out, "I'm so mad. Do you really think he paid it off?"

Kate says, "God, you think that could have been, what Tweets, like, ninety-thousand? Did he have that kinda' money?"

Mom responds, "Hell if I know, shit, I obviously don't know anything this man did."

I look at him and squeeze the cold metal rails, "You have me so mad, Dad. I have never been so angry with you. You could die any second, and you know what I think?"

My hands go up in the air, accompanied by an obnoxious groan. Kate and Mom laugh. Kate shouts, "Oh my God, you are so funny."

I laugh too, and once again we can't control ourselves. Mom gets up and grabs her crotch, "Oh shit, I have to pee. God dammit, Molly, I'm going to pee my pants."

She runs for the bathroom. I am kneeling down on the floor next to the bed, holding my stomach. I open my eyes, and see the bucket with a full bag of pee.

"Shit, his pee is full."

I put on gloves and begin the task. I say loudly, "Hey Dad, I'm emptying your pee bag. Did Claire ever empty your pee bag?"

"No, only his wallet!" Kate shouts.

Mom's laugh echoes through the wall.

Finally we calm down. Mom is on the mattress again, and Kate and I each on a couch.

Mom is fast asleep as Kate flips through the channels.

Within minutes, Kate is asleep, and now I flip through the channels. My stomach is sore from laughing, but it really isn't funny. I try to evoke my fury, but I am too tired. I turn off the television and fall asleep.

Today his gallery does not cheer him on, instead, taunts his errors, and asks for some excuse for his bad play. Even though I know if we finish, we win, I don't want to carry his bag anymore. Maybe I'm not the one who should. He never shared his winnings with me, yet his most important victory is near, and I'm the one who coaches him.

A distant noise brings me out of a trance and back to the living room. It's Mom laughing.

"Kate, is she awake?" I sit up and ask.

Kate yawns, "I don't know what she's doing."

We lie back down and close our eyes. Mom continues to giggle.

She calls out, "I'm laughing. I realized something while I was asleep."

"What's that?" Kate asks.

Mom can barely get her words out before she bursts into laughter again, "If he did pay it off, that means he paid off her mortgage, and never paid off mine. We still have a mortgage on this house. What an asshole!"

He starts breathing heavily.

"Maybe he is trying to tell us something?" I say.

Mom says, "Oh Richard, I can't believe you, what did you really do?"

The clock says 3:06, as we cuddle up in our blankets and discuss the situation, again.

I fade off, hearing Kate's voice in the distance, "Claire had a lot of people convinced. She was very devious. Dad fell into her web."

Mom replies, but I do not hear her words. I allow myself to fall into a dream.

Day 45

The door opens with a knock and Babe walks in, "Hello, I have been calling all morning and the phone is busy."

Kate is the first to respond, "What time is it?"

Babe replies, "It's nine-thirty. What happened last night?"

Mom's head pops out to where Babe can see it, "He paid off her mortgage, and didn't even pay off mine."

Laughter immediately follows, as she gets up, grabs her crotch, and runs down the hallway.

I say, "How about I make us some Bloody Marys?"

Kate gets up quickly, "Yeah, sounds good."

"What are all these papers?" Babe asks as she steps over them, making her way to Dad.

She yells out louder, "Hello, can you guys hear me? What the hell's going on?"

"Hey, you want a Bloody Mary?" I ask Babe.

"Appears, I do. Now, how is he doing?"

"He has pretty much been asleep since Friday," I tell her.

Mom walks back out, and asks Babe, "Where were you guys last night?"

"Grandkids had a play."

"Well, you missed a hell of a night."

"I can tell. What happened?"

They sit down at the table, and Mom tells the weekend of Claire, in great detail. I finish making the drinks. I serve them, and say, "Here's to Claire's mortgage."

We raise our glasses, and in slow motion, clink.

Kate says, "Oh my God. This is so good. I hope you have plenty of this."

"Actually, that's the last of the mix," I confess.

"Don't worry, we have a bunch at the house," Babe offers. "I will call Henry."

"Oh, there's Henry now," I say, as Wrigley runs up the deck steps.

I open the patio door, and Wrigley bursts in, full throttle.

"Hey Henry, Babe says you have Bloody Mary mix at the house."

"Go get it, sweetie," Babe yells out. "We're going to need it."

"Boy, must be good news. I will be right back."

He darts through the living room and out the front door. Kate and Babe are already finished with their drinks. I begin to sing, "One life, one love, let's get together and feel all right."

I continue the lyrics as I get up, and run to the stairs. Wrigley chases after me. I jump halfway, but tumble to the bottom. "Shit that hurt. Fuck!"

I have never missed that jump.

After a quick few puffs of Mary Jane, I'm back upstairs. Everyone is laughing, as Mom repeats the weekend's events.

"We need our drinks refreshed," Kate hollers at me.

I grab the new bottle of mix from the table, and go to the counter to make another round.

"Have you asked Dick if it's true?" Babe asks. "Maybe he will give you a sign."

Kate and I make eye contact then run to the bed. I grab his hand, and say, "Okay Dad, I know we have been upset, but we need to know some things. Please try to answer these questions. Squeeze my hand if you paid off Claire's mortgage."

We all wait, hoping this could actually work, but unfortunately nothing happens.

Babe suggests, "Start small. Just say words until he responds."

Kate hands me my drink. I sip it and try to think of what word could get his attention. After almost finishing it, I hand her the glass. "Okay, here we go. Dad, I'm going to say a bunch of names. If any of these names are significant, or something we should know about, please squeeze my hand."

I increase my volume as I begin to list, "Curtis…Mom…Kate…Claire."

I feel a movement in my hand, "Oh my God, I think he did something."

"Do it again," Kate yells.

"Okay Dad, let's try again," I continue, "Kate…Molly…Mom…Claire."

I feel another slight pressure in my palm, "I really think he is responding to her name."

"Molls, will you make me another drink?" Mom asks.

I give up, and go to the kitchen.

"I'm telling you, when I said her name he responded."

Mom replies, "These drinks are very strong, and I think you have had a little bit—"

The sound of the front door opening stops her words. We all freeze.

Pastor's voice fills the room, "Sounds like a party in here."

We let out a sigh and laugh. I approach the table to hand Mom her drink. She says, "The Pastor is here, the Pastor is here. Hi Pastor."

She gets up and attempts to explain the circumstance, "Last night, we got some interesting news, and well, we have had a rough night and morning from it."

"I can see that," Pastor replies. "Well, how is Richard doing?"

"He's been out since Friday," Mom answers.

"It's like he knew exactly when this would all go down," I add. "His timing on this is perfect. We can't even confront him and find out the truth."

"What exactly did you find out?" Pastor says in a low voice.

Mom starts the story again. Kate whispers in my ear, "Make me another one."

"No, not while he is here."

"She is nowhere near the end. I won't make it through this story again without a drink."

Within seconds, Kate gets up and goes to the fridge. I watch her pull out the orange juice, get a new glass, fill it with ice, and then pour vodka in it. Mom finally finishes the saga; Pastor just smiles and says, "Let's go pray with Richard."

With effort we get up and gather around the bed, grabbing one another's arms.

Pastor prays something about Richard being ready for the Kingdom and guiding his family to understanding, as we concentrate on remaining upright, until finally, *Amen.*

Babe, using the bedrails to hold herself up, says, "Let's say the Lord's Prayer."

Pastor begins again, "Our Father…"

We say it the best we can, but mostly slurs come out. Babe is the worst. She is a couple of words behind us, getting louder, and less understandable with each phrase.

We finish this time with a bunch of jagged *Amens.*

Pastor says, "Okay, I have to get back to the church. You should probably get some rest."

We sit in awkward silence until Pastor is in the driveway. Mom says, "That's just great. He comes over here, and we're blitzed out of our minds."

I laugh, and then everyone joins in.

"It's not funny," Mom yells. "It's only ten in the morning."

"Oh Tweets, think about your mortgage," Kate says.

"What an asshole," Mom shouts.

We are back at the table and now all singing, "One love, one life, let's get together and feel all right."

Babe and Henry are dancing. I take a pile of cards and spread them out on the table. There are four decks scattered in front of me. I take my time mixing them up. My fingers move over the slippery cool tops, making circles, covering the table. I say, "All right, who thinks I can pick a four?"

"A four?" Kate replies.

"Yeah, a four."

My hand goes into the middle, somewhere deep, and slides a single card, with my middle finger, to the end of the table. I flip it over, and the four of hearts is on the other side.

"No way!" Kate shouts.

I yell, "Hey, Babe, you think I can pull a seven?"

Babe turns around from Henry's arm, and stumbles over to me. She grabs the chair, as she falls into it, and says, "I'll shit if you do."

"All right, get ready to shit yourself 'cause here we go."

All eyes are on my middle finger, hovering over the cards, but this time it goes to the left and picks out one from a loner pile. I slide it to Babe.

"Could it be?" I ask.

I bring it to my face and flip it. I see it with my own two eyes first.

I can't believe it.

I slam it on the table. The seven of diamonds stares out at everybody.

Mom screams out, "Oh my God! Molly, how did you

do that?"

"I have no idea. I was just joking around. I didn't know it would happen."

"But you did know it would happen, or you wouldn't have tried it," Kate says.

I take the two cards and balance them for display on a shelf against the wall. "Now the number will always be looking at us."

*

It's quiet, as I cuddle up on the couch, dozing. Mom is taking a shower and Kate is getting dressed.

Heather comes in the front door. "I'm so sorry to be late," she announces.

I respond, "Oh yeah, that's right. Amy never came this morning."

Heather replies, "No, I was supposed to be here. I'm so sorry, how is he doing?"

"He is still asleep."

"Still no response?"

"Not really, he has been out cold."

Kate walks in, falls into her spot, and covers her legs with the blanket.

Heather says, "Well, his vitals aren't too bad, but he is fading faster than he was."

She leans into us, and whispers, "I would say by Wednesday."

Mom enters the Scene.

"Hi Tweedy, how are you?" Heather says.

"Well, we have had quite a weekend."

She repeats the Claire story, and exactly thirty-eight minutes later finishes with, "The Pastor was here and we were drinking *at ten in the morning!*"

Heather asks, "He never told you about any money he gave her?"

Mom replies, "No."

"Well, that is beside the point anyway. The doctor put him in hospice because he is dying," Heather says. "This is the process of death. If Claire can't understand that, then she doesn't need to be a part of it. She is not someone you need here in this time of distress. She is obviously mentally unstable. Don't let her in your house. Meet her outside, tell her that it's your house, and you can't have her negativity around."

"I can do that?" Mom asks.

"Of course you can," she declares. "He is your husband, and this is your house. She has no right to be here if you don't want her here. I will personally call her and tell her, as his nurse, it is best at this time, if she doesn't come back. You guys don't need this right now. It's just too much."

She continues, "You are about to lose your husband after long months of suffering. When that bed is gone; you will mourn its existence. All the attention is on her right now. Screw her. Don't let her around. We are close, but it's not over yet. Don't let her in the house."

She walks out the door. Mom says, "Heather is serious. She seemed really upset about all this."

"It's good to know the hospice place knows Claire is mentally unstable," Kate adds.

"Yeah, sounds like she can't do much as far as the assisted suicide thing goes," I reply.

"Oh, that's just crazy," Kate replies. "Her saying that alone, proves she's nuts."

"I hope no one else comes, I really want to take a nap," Mom says.

"Well, go in your room, and shut the door," I suggest. "You need to sleep."

She grabs her pillow, "Okay, but wake me up if something happens."

"I need to go take a shower," I say to Kate.

"Okay, I will keep an eye on the mortgage payer."

Mom's voice pierces through the walls from her room, "He never paid my mortgage. Mortgage payer, my ass."

Once again, we laugh. I grab my crotch, run to the stairs, and yell out, "Shit, now, I'm gonna' pee my pants."

The smell of the hard water is inviting as I rotate my head under the spigot. My mind is racing.

He never gave me anything. Not one thing that I can remember. Mom always did, but never Dad.

My back hits the shower glass, hard. I slide down and my ass hits the floor. My head goes in my knees; I sob. I wake up choking on the water, not knowing how much time has passed.

I get up and get ready to go back upstairs, back to The Scene. I hear voices as I turn toward the living room. Chloe is here. She says, "Hey Molls."

I sit down beside her as she continues her conversation with Kate.

Dad coughs. Kate, Chloe, and I run to his side. "Oh my God, this is the first thing he has done since Friday," I shout.

Kate says, "Dad, can you hear me?"

His hand trembles forward and one eyelid shivers lightly.

"He is trying to open his eye," Chloe yells.

It pops open. The eyeball is large, blue, and limp. I whisper to him, "Hey Dad, hey. Dad, we are here. Can you see me?"

The lid falls suddenly; he doesn't have the strength to keep it up.

Kate says, "You better call Heather. The hospice book says they open their eye right before the end."

I run to the phone and dial. I say into the phone, "Hey Heather, it's Molly, he just opened one eye and then it closed."

"Really? I'll come back, that's a sign."

Kate is holding his hand and begging, "Dad, please squeeze my hand. Squeeze my hand, Dad. Come on Dad, squeeze my hand."

She finally gives up, and neatly puts his hand back in the bed. She says, "I need a glass of wine."

"Oh, can I have one?" Chloe asks.

Mom's voice from the hallway is soft, "I'll have a Bailey's."

"Hi Tweets, you get a nice nap?" Chloe gets up, and embraces Mom.

"Chloe, where were you last night? Your mother wanted to spend the night here," Mom says.

Chloe laughs, "Oh my God, that would have been awful, just awful."

The three of them clink their drinks. Kate says to Mom,

"Tweets, Dad opened his eye."

Mom yells out, "What? He did?"

She runs to him and says, "Oh Richard, can you hear me?"

Our eyes fix on him, for we think he will die at any moment. We have thought this for days, weeks, even months, but we still hope to be there for the last heartbeat.

A few minutes later, Heather walks through the door, "How is he?"

"He is out again," I reply.

She checks him. "His heart rate is very low, and his breathing is much lighter since earlier."

Leslie opens the door, and asks, "Is everything okay? All the cars made me think..."

Mom says, "He is failing."

Heather leans into us, "I would think by morning."

She sits down cross-legged in the middle of the floor. Kate asks her, "Have you always worked in hospice."

"I actually started in the labor room of the maternity ward. After holding the hand of a new life entering the world, I wanted to hold someone's hand that was leaving the earth as well. I wanted to experience both situations."

I reply, "Wow! That is crazy."

Chloe says, "Do you like one more than the other."

She replies, "I think this is much more rewarding for me, but both are like nothing I can explain."

We spend the next couple hours learning about each other, and conversing about simple things.

*

Leslie is the last to leave, and asks, "Are you sure you don't want me to stay?"

Mom replies, "If you want to that's fine, but you don't have to, the girls and I will be all right."

She says, "Okay, but call me as soon as—"

Mom interrupts, "I will, I will."

She shuts and locks the door. She turns back around, and says, "I'm turning all the lights off too. I'm tired, and I don't want anyone else coming in."

Within minutes we are curled up in our spots asleep.

His breathing fades away and I wake up. I listen for the sound of his breath because I know it is the last sound. I'm up at his side, staring at his chest, but I can't tell if it is moving.

"What's going on?" Kate asks.

"I thought he stopped breathing, but I think he is now."

"Well, is he?"

I see his chest rise, and hear the breath once more. "Yes, he is breathing. He is fine."

"Oh yeah, I can hear him now. He did stop, didn't he?"

"I don't know, sounded like it, it woke me up."

Day 46

A loud pounding registers in my head. My eyes come out of darkness, and squint at the light.

Mom's voice is loud, "Shit, I locked the door last night."

She stomps by me, and opens the door.

"Oh, it's Amy. Thank God."

"Good morning," Amy says with a bubbly intonation.

I head over to the bed, and pull out a pair of gloves. I begin to peel off the tape.

Amy says, "We have to change his sheets today, too."

I reply, "Really, even now."

She responds, "He could lie here another week."

Mom walks up, and begins to straighten up the medical objects on the table, "You think by looking at him, he could last another week?"

Amy studies his body. Her fingers press on his chest and outer area of the tumor.

I pull the gauze out from the inner hole, and scream,

"Oh God, the smell is awful."

I turn and gag. I grab a paper towel and spit in it.

Amy says, "Here, put this under your nose."

She grabs a jar of Vicks from her bag.

The tumor has all its colors today. The tissue around the sides is dead, brown, and dry. The main core is an emerald bubble with dark red blotches.

Amy hands me the last piece of tape. I ask, "Well, what do you think?"

"I just don't know. Heather called me last night and said to double-check my phone this morning, because she thought he would be gone by now. It's impossible to say."

She pauses then says, "Okay, I'm going to bathe him, and then we will do the sheets. Before we start, I have to tell you, putting him on his side could cause his heart to stop."

Kate gets off her couch, stretching, "So he could die, like right now?"

"Yes, it's not likely, but it could happen."

As we roll him, Mom says, "Man, he is heavy."

The four of us struggle, more than any other time he has been rolled, and most times have been just Mom and me. He is completely dead weight. After a lot of huffing and puffing, he is back in position. His breathing is still constant, but his color is light purple and his face is drawn-in.

I watch Amy gather her things.

Will this be the last time I see her?

"Bye, see you Thursday," she says, as she walks out the door.

The phone rings and Mom goes to answer. Kate and I look in the fridge.

"I have to warn you, he is really bad. I don't know if it would be good, if he saw him," Mom says into the phone.

"I wonder who that is," I say to Kate.

Mom responds, "All right. Yeah, that's fine. We will see you soon."

She hangs up the phone.

Kate asks, "They are coming, now?"

"They will be here in about twenty minutes."

I yell out, "Who?"

Mom replies quietly, "Riffling and Fran. Fran says Riffling is adamant about seeing Dad right now. I could hear him screaming at her. He was saying, 'I have to see Weasel.' So I thought, screw it."

Kate and I wait, eagerly. We wonder why Dirk wants to see Dad so suddenly. Mom is in the kitchen, wiping down the sink, when the door opens.

Dirk is leaning over, grunting for breath. I meet him at the door, and say, "Hey Dirk. Here, grab my arm."

We walk to where the carpet begins, and he says, "I got it from here."

With his claw cane he approaches The Scene. He grabs the steal rail with one hand. "Hey Weasel, it's me, Dirk. I just came from the doctor's office. We got in the car, and I said to Fran that I had to come see you right now."

He pauses, and grabs the drawstring from his pants with his other hand. He tightens the string around his fist. "We had a lot of years together, buddy, almost our whole lives. Since we were kids, we been friends. I guess, when it's time, it's time. Bye, Dick. Goodbye."

His head falls a bit, as his hand squeezes the rail tighter. He grabs his cane, turns, and sighs, "Come on Fran, let's go home."

She replies, "That's it? We just got here."

"I'm done, it's time to go."

"Okay, fine by me. I'm sorry, Tweedy, for the interruption, but I guess we're leaving now."

Mom hugs her, and says, "No problem. I'm glad Dirk got to see him."

*

Chloe is sitting at the dining room table, as I walk out from the office.

I approach her and say, "What's up?"

She replies, "Hey, why is there a four and seven on the shelf up there?"

"Yesterday I picked them from the deck; it was crazy. I will demonstrate what happened."

I take my hands and begin to circle the cards still scattered on the table. "Okay, I said I was going to pick a four, and I put my hand in, and I picked a four."

I put my hand in the pile and bring out a card. I turn it over, and slam it on the table. It is the four of hearts. I scream, "Oh my God, that's crazy. I did it again!"

Chloe replies, "No fucking way. You're messing with me."

Kate says, "No, she did it yesterday, too."

"Okay, let's see if I can pick the seven."

My middle finger circles the cards and finally slides one to the end of the table. I grab it and throw it down, "No, just an eight."

Chloe says, "An eight. Close enough."

I grab the two cards and put them on the shelf between the other two.

*

Kate and I sit on the floor with piles of paper, and once again try to find proof of Dad's secret.

I ask, "I wonder what else we don't know?"

Kate replies, "Yeah, I've been thinking that, too."

Mom yells, "Don't say that. I don't need anyone showing up here claiming to be his son."

Kate replies, "I know it's crazy, but I thought the same thing."

I join in, "Well if he does, we will send him to Claire to get his father's money."

Kate interrupts, "Claire always got what she wanted. He spent a lot of money on her, more than he ever spent on Curtis or me. He said he was going to buy me my first car. He traded in the family car to get my car. It was my car for about two days, and then it became the family car. I was so mad at him."

Mom replies, "That sounds just like your dad."

Kate continues, "Then one day, he said he needed to take it to work, but him and his buddies went to the track. I went into work at the Avenue, and he wasn't there. He met his friends earlier, and they all left in my car."

"Track, like horse racing?" I ask.

"Oh yeah, he loved to bet on the horses."

"What? He despised gambling," I argue.

"No. He loved going to the track."

"Not the Dad I know. What the hell happened?"

"I don't know. I forgot about it till now," Kate answers.

Mom shakes her head, and flips through a magazine, "Who is this man?"

A few quiet moments go by. We are all trying to understand the situation.

I ask Kate, "What about his drinking? Did he drink, a lot, all the time?"

She replies, "Yeah, he did. Some nights he would sit at the bar with Uncle Buck, and go through a couple bottles of booze."

"Booze?" I scream. "He only drinks beer."

Kate chuckles back, "Beer? Well, he drank hard liquor when he was younger."

"What kind?" I ask.

"Seagram's Seven."

"Straight?"

"No, with Coke."

"That's crazy. I have never seen him drink a drop of hard liquor. It was always beer."

"Well, after the car accident when Curtis and Claire were hurt, he promised he would never drink again. I'm pretty sure that's when he switched to beer."

Mom smirks, "Sounds like Dad. What an asshole. Like, going from liquor to beer is 'not drinking.' Beer was all he drank, and he was drunk all the time."

He lies in his living room, helpless, hearing his sins revealed to the ones he betrayed. These hours must be important for his soul to free.

Day 47

Mom went to see her financial guy, so it's just me and Kate. Dad seems better today. His face is plump again and has color. The skeleton look is gone; there is a bag full of pee.

Kate is occupying herself by looking through the pantry, "Look at the date of this peanut butter—seven years old."

"He asked Pastor how he could go to Heaven," I say. "He was worried about his sins."

Kate laughs, "He should have been."

"Oh my God, look!" she yells.

His face is twitching frantically. I follow Kate, as she runs to him, "Oh my God, his eye!"

The blue glaze hits my heart, as it shines past his wilted lid. I kneel down, and whisper, "Hi Dad."

He whispers back, "Hi."

His eyelid falls heavily, and the moment is over.

I wet a swab and put it on his lips, trying to coax another word from his breath.

Only a few moments have past, when the same eye flutters.

"He just mouthed, *I love you*," Kate says.

The eyelid is frail and deteriorated, but the blue of his eye is unbelievably bright.

The core of the eye represents his soul. It has seen the glory, and it is glazed with intense beauty.

His face is twitching again. I lean into him, and say, "You can go Dad. We will be okay, and take care of each other."

I look at Kate and she nods at me to continue. I stroke his hair, "I'm sure your family in Heaven will be much saner."

Kate chuckles. I try to be serious, and continue in a comforting tone, "Claire will be fine, too. She is just having a difficult time accepting it."

Kate says, "Look at his expression when you said her name."

I grab his hand and say, "Okay, Dad, if you are worried about Mom, make a face."

He has no movement.

I say, "If you are worried about Curtis make a face."

Still, he has no response.

I raise my eyebrows, look at Kate, and say to him, "If you are worried about Claire, make a face."

His face twists into a grimace. I rub his hand and say, "It is okay Dad. I'm sorry, I didn't mean to upset you."

His face is locked in that frightening expression. Twenty minutes go by.

"He looks really upset," Kate says.

"Yeah, I'm going to call hospice."

Courtney asks me, "Is it like a grimace look?"

"Exactly."

"He is agitated by something. You need to give him the drops, now."

Within a few minutes, his face has relaxed. His eyelid is wiggling again, trying to open.

I hear the back door, and yell, "Mom, come here, quick!"

She runs in and says, "What?"

"Look at his eye. It is going to open."

She sees it flutter, and says, "Richard, we are fine. We are all here, well, most of us. We will be okay—well, most of us."

"Mom, stop it!" I shout.

Mom walks back to the kitchen.

"I am going to take a shower," Kate says.

I am sitting next to him, waiting for something. His eye opens, and he notices me. I yell out, "Oh my God!"

Kate runs out, and says, "Dad, hi."

"Mom, come here, quick," I yell again.

She screams back, "I'm going to the bathroom."

"Mom, now! His eye is open."

She runs out to his side, "Oh Pa, Pa, it's okay."

His eye slowly shuts again. Mom turns to walk away. I say, "Mom, wait."

She replies, "I have to finish going potty."

I say to Dad, "You saw Mom. Wasn't that nice?"

Kate chuckles.

"Only in this house," I say. "His eye is open again!"

Mom runs out, "It's okay Richard, you did what you thought was right. You can go now. Everything will be fine."

She stands up to walk away again.

"Mom, can't you just chill for one moment?"

"I have stuff in the car I need to bring in."

I say, "There you go. You got to see Mom. See, everything is fine, Dad."

The blue glow is slowly covered by its limp cap, and for the last time I see sunlight recede from his sight.

Mom flits from one thing to another and won't rest. I finally yell out, "Mom, you need to sit down."

"I can't sit down, I'm busy."

"You need to because of the stress and your heart."

I hear the back door open, as she leaves in the middle of our conversation.

Over an hour later she sits in her chair and says, "I'm ready to rest."

"You should be," I say.

"Yeah, on the way home today, I fell asleep in the car on Big Lumber Road."

"What?" Kate screams. "Tweets, that's why you need to relax, this is too much stress."

*

Another night has come. Kate is at the bed, checking on

him. She lifts up the blanket and says, "Look at this."

I approach. Deep, dark blue and purple blotches cover his feet and legs, like a five year old painted them.

Is this the start of another stage?

I work on the computer, but my eyes are getting weary. I walk out to the living room. His breathing is the lightest I've seen.

"We need to do the tumor," Kate says.

"Okay."

I fixate on it, examining the squishy discolored hole and its surroundings. I've done this every day, and some days twice. I watched it change shape, size, and color many times. I am almost sickened, knowing this is the end. This is the last time I will run this routine.

I take my time. I have become good at the task. I am proud to be able to do it, and saddened that it will stop. I brush my hand against his clammy cheek. The back of my hand grazes his nose and it feels like ice.

"Holy shit," I say to Kate. "Feel his nose."

She presses her finger to his nose, and says, "Wow, that is cold."

Death is cold. It is gradually overcoming his body.

Does it spread from his nose? How much longer will it take?

I walk back into the office and sit down, but I can't concentrate. Something doesn't seem right.

It is a few minutes after 11:00 p.m.

How many more days can this go on? I know he is ready now. It took a while, but he figured it out. I guess it's a miracle. Love destroying fear in the final days, to uplift his soul to what he knows as Heaven. I imagine Dad's entrance at the wedding.

He will celebrate, and be part of all that is true, but he is missing something – his innocence.

I dart through the house into the laundry room, turn the light on, and close the door. There it is. It reminds me of a wedding dress: white, and about to start a brand new journey. I wrap my hand around its soft, plush threads, and say, "Okay, it's time for you to do your thing. Show's on."

I take long, powerful strides back to the bed.

"I'm not crazy, I just want to try something," I say to Kate, who is on a couch facing the bed.

"Okay," she replies.

Taking the blanket completely off of him, I say, "Dad, I have something for you. It's the white robe. Can you feel it Dad? It's nice and soft."

I drape it over his entire body, and rub it against his arm.

I take the brush from the table that holds the utensils of the past few weeks. It feels like I am combing the hair of a doll. His hair doesn't even seem real. It is thick and curvy. I can remember brushing it when I was a young girl.

"Now your hair is nice and combed. You look real spiffy Dad, just like you always did. You can go to sleep now. You can go home."

The robe glistens, as I kiss his forehead, and whisper, "I love you, Dad."

He looks content. His face is full, and for the first time he truly looks like the Dad I remember.

It's almost midnight when I walk back into the office. I sit down and my head falls into my hands. My fingers interlace, and I begin to talk to God, "I have to put all my faith in the white robe. Please Lord, he is ready for you. He is prepared. Take him home. Please, just take him home. He wants to go and be with you. I am asking for a miracle, I know, but please take him tonight. I will be a better person. I already am because of this. I have learned patience. I saw love destroy fear. I saw him battle his past life and reach out for his future life, and I realize that's what life is, a fight, but it's worth the result, in Heaven. End his struggle, Lord. Please."

I'm breathing hard and my heart is racing. As I inhale, I feel a presence. Peace and harmony surround me.

My hands unfold. I get up and walk back out into The Scene. My mattress is available tonight. Kate is on the couch and Mom is in her room. It's now 12:20 a.m. I lie down beside the brown metal frame.

Kate and I fill the room with giggles as we discuss Dad. Two daughters waiting with their dying father and satisfying his mortal being with laughter, must be considered a good farewell. His breathing sometimes becomes too quiet, I watch, and after a few seconds the robe rises once more.

It is 2:30 a.m., the room is silent, and sleep takes us.

My eyes open, and I peek up at him. I don't see the robe move, but I know it is okay.

It's time to rest.

I fall back asleep.

Day 48

Kate's voice is loud, waking me, "Molly, Molly."

I whisper, "Yeah?"

"He's not breathing."

My upper body rises in military style. I turn toward the picture I have feared for so long and see Kate's hand on his chest.

"He's not breathing," she repeats, shaking her head.

I move my eyes to view his face; it is frozen, immovable, stuck, without life.

"All right, I better get Mom."

I stand. "Oh my God, the robe!"

Kate replies, "I know."

I pace back and forth.

Why, after all these days, did I remember its existence only last night?

Kate is motionless, with her hand on his chest.

A few moments go by, and I say, "Shit, I need to get Mom."

I walk down the hallway and see myself as a young girl, running to my room. As many times as I have traveled this hall, I never thought this would be a walk I would take.

I enter her room. "Mom, he's gone," I say, with surprising calmness.

She jumps up, "He is? No, is he?"

"He's gone."

She runs out to The Scene, and whimpers out, "Oh Richard. Is he really gone?"

Kate has not moved, but she responds to Mom's cry, "Yeah, he is."

Mom shouts out, "Oh my God, the robe! When did you do that?"

"Last night."

She repeats, "Last night. Oh my God, he has the robe on."

Her fingers stroke it. "Why did you do that?"

"I don't know, I guess it was time."

I am frantically pacing around the entire room, "I guess I should call hospice."

Kate replies, "Yeah, he still is not breathing."

Even though we know he is dead, we are not in the moment of realization.

I dial the number, but hit the wrong digits. The buttons 8-4-7 elude my unsteady fingers. I try three times before I get it right.

"Hi, Courtney, it's Molly. He's gone."

"I'm so sorry. Is everyone okay?" she replies.

"Yeah, I think so. Are you going to come out?"

"I will be there in about 45 minutes."

Kate's hand is still glued to his chest.

Mom is in the kitchen, waking people up, giving them the news they have been waiting for.

So this is it? This is how it played out? The picture is not as drastic as I assumed it would be.

Kate is standing at his bedside, the palm of her hand is spread out on his heart. His heart, covered by the cloth of the white robe that warmed him as he ended this round and entered his banquet of Heaven.

To live eighty years and get away with so many lies and secrets that affected so many people was an accomplishment. That is until he was told he had a month to live. His response was, "I'm in big trouble, aren't I?"

Golf is one of the few sports played at all ages, especially the later years. A golfer who has played throughout life realizes that youth and strength go together. The speed of the golf swing relates to the distance the ball travels – the faster, the farther. With length, corners are cut and obstacles are almost invisible. Time decreases power, and eventually the hazards come into play. Age forces us to take the turns. The course becomes harder and longer, accuracy becomes everything. Keeping the body healthy and in good physical shape is a lifelong test. However, it's the spirit, the mind, the love, the fear, and the desire that force us to make the final putt.

Mom, on the phone, keeps repeating the phrase, "He is gone."

The door opens and Babe and Henry enter the death-filled room. Babe, with hesitation, walks up to the bed, "He has on the robe."

Her hand glides over its lushness. She turns and looks at me in astonishment.

"I put it on him last night."

She turns around and walks to the kitchen. She embraces Mom, "How are you doing?"

"I'm okay, just trying to call everyone. Did you see the robe?"

"Yes, I did. What happened?"

"I don't know. I was in bed."

Lynn comes through the door. She hugs me, and says, "I'm so sorry, sweetie."

She approaches the body as though it was a throne. She too slides her hand along the white cloth.

Dad's face is already different. The color is changing. The skeletal frame is back and more precise.

Leslie walks in. She embraces me, saying, "He finally went."

She moves toward the bed and says, "Oh, you have the robe on him."

Her fingers spread through its folds.

My father is lying dead just feet away from me. The room is filled with people, as dusk turns into day.

Courtney asks, "Do you mind if I wash him down a little?"

I reply, "No, that's fine."

I am sitting on the mattress facing everyone. Their faces are sober and weary from an early rise. I am thankful dawn is here, and light finally shines through the darkness of what appeared to be an endless night.

Courtney is standing at the table of utensils, and asks, "Do you want to keep any of this?"

I reply, "No, get rid of it all."

She picks up the wastebasket and begins to clear the debris. She says, "The funeral representative will be here in about thirty minutes. Would you like me to wait?"

I reply, "No. We are fine. Go ahead. Thank you for everything."

We circle the bed in prayer for the last time. So many different arms have wrapped this bed. The final hands as they intertwine: Mom, Nate, Chloe, Kate, Lynn, Leslie, Aunt Susan, Henry, Babe, Pastor, and Me. I hear nothing of the prayer.

It's over. His body will be gone. This bed will be gone. I will be gone.

Amen, drones off all tongues, as we break the ring.

Pastor says, "We already have a visitation and funeral scheduled Monday and Tuesday. We will have to have to have Dick's funeral on Wednesday."

Mom says, "That's fine."

After a moment she screams, "Geez and crackers! Wednesday? Do you know what day Wednesday is?"

My mind is muddled. She yells, "Wednesday is the seventh, his funeral is going to be on 4-7."

Pastor smiles, "Now, that's just a coincidence, don't worry about it."

Today is April 1st and also Maundy Thursday; this is a significant day.

*

I stand at his head, and stroke my fingers through his hair. It is so soft and thick. It's hard to believe it rests on the head of a corpse.

"She didn't throw it all away."

I walk over to the table in a rage, and scream, "Does this look like everything is gone?"

I throw all the remaining medical crap in the garbage. As I bend down to pick up an errant shot, I see a familiar object. It's the end of a bamboo-handled back scratcher that has always been in the magazine rack next to his chair. I can't stop the tears from leaving my eyes. I slowly turn around, amazed by its value, and say, "When I was a kid he would scratch this on my arm, and then I would do his. He loved it. I loved it."

Two ladies walk through the door and say they are from the funeral home.

These two little women are going to haul him out of here? I guess big guys are not always the answer to moving something. I helped move a soul to glory, and I'm not very big at all.

The last moment is here and I can't bear it. I lose all strength, and fall to my knees, ridiculously weeping and gasping for air. Chloe is quick to comfort me.

I cry, "I'm sorry, I'm losing it."

She replies, "You don't have to apologize."

We kneel together at the side of the man who gave us life, but now is gone from his own.

Tears fall in the house that prepared him. However, in the house that holds him now, tears do not exist.

I don't want to look like an idiot, so I hobble back onto my feet, only to become absorbed in his hair, stroking it. The two women wait patiently. I say to him, "You look really good Dad. You really do."

In slow motion, I press my lips against his forehead.

"Goodbye," I whisper to him.

My fingers glide through his curls, "I'm just so obsessed with his hair."

The funeral lady asks, "Would you like a lock of it?"

I reply, "No, that's okay."

I finally let go, and say, "Okay, you can take him."

Mom isn't even in the room; she is outside.

I stand at the head of the bed; my hand could reach his yellowish skin. I am stuck to their every move, as they glide him onto a board, and easily lift him onto the gurney covered with the body bag. They gently slip him into the bag. It's not black, like a garbage bag. His is beautiful; it is maroon with sparkles, and made of a heavy fabric like the cloth of a curtain. They did the task with much caution. I was on them like a hawk, not missing a move. They carefully zip it up to his neck, and then wheel him toward the door. I walk beside his head, watching it jiggle around. Everyone follows right behind me. The gallery is full. Many people stand on the grass.

We make our way through the crowd, and the sun hits my face like water to a wilted rose. The light glistens off the glitter of the cloth that wraps his diseased body. The zipper slowly evaporates his face and they slide him into the van.

I stand in the driveway and wave, as they pull away.

Pretty good send off for a Dick.

What he did is now irrelevant. It doesn't matter how many mistakes he made, or how many shots it took him. What counts is that he played. He completed the round, as difficult as it was. He ended life and suffered death. I think his score was high, his agony a bit much, for the actual game he played. In my opinion, his life didn't deserve an aching death, but then again, I was just his caddie. He was the one swinging the club.

We sit in thought, not sure what to do next.

I say, "I can't believe it was 47 days since I got here."

Aunt Susan replies, "Well, technically, it was 48."

I shrug my shoulders and say, "Close enough."

Aunt Susan's face freezes. Chloe looks at me with the same surprised expression.

*

Chloe and I are on our way back from the store. We pull in the driveway. The garage door is open. I can see Mom standing at the kitchen counter. Growing up, in the summer, the garage and the back door were always open. Anyone and everyone would walk right in. Since I have been here, the garage door has been closed, and all fans have entered through the front door. Coming in from this view, I do not see it right away, but a bit of death is still there when I turn the corner.

I ask Mom, "Why is that still here?"

She replies, "They called and said they are overloaded, but they hope to be here by five."

"That bed can't be here tonight, it needs to be gone," I storm downstairs.

*

It's just after noon when I make our first batch of

drinks. Mom shouts from the hall, "Here are all the pictures."

She walks out with a pile of albums, "Oh, and let me get the collage off the wall downstairs."

After a few hours of looking through pictures, I can't focus anymore, so I make my way to the office.

I hear Chloe's voice, "I think he's here."

I get up and run out to the bed, one final time.

Kate makes her way to the door. She says, "Hi, you made it."

His voice has a bit of a drawl as he says, "Yeah, it's been crazy. Last minute set ups all day, this is my first take down."

He is my age, a little short, with an athletic build, and a rugged, yet, innocent face. Kate, Chloe, and I sit down to watch him take the brown frame apart.

He is cautious in handling the components of the crib. He uses a screwdriver to detach the parts, carefully piling the pieces of the frame, without clatter.

I am amazed at how precisely he does his task. For just a bed, he treats it with great respect. The bed was dismantled just like the life that had lain in it—piece by piece, examined, and perfectly prepared. The Scene dissolves.

Those rails met many hands connected to the soul that was within them. The rails protected him, allowing him to go home.

We stare at the empty space.

Kate says, "We need to change the room around; make it completely different."

Kate and I move the furniture, and within minutes we have the room upside down.

Mom runs in from the laundry room, whispering, "Claire is here. Claire is here."

Claire walks through the back door and turns toward

us. Kate robotically embraces her sibling. I continue to rearrange the room.

Claire asks, "What are you guys doing?"

"We need a different look," I say.

With a snide giggle, she replies, "Well, I hope you don't throw your back out. That can be very painful, I know."

What the fuck does that have to do with anything?

Luckily, Bridgett and Blake walk in. Bridgett hugs me as she whispers in my ear, "I'm so sorry, and I mean, for everything. I mean everything."

It's late and Curtis is drunk. Nate is holding him up as he slurs dramatically, "Dad is dead, dead. My dad is dead."

Kate and I follow Nate as he maneuvers him out to the car through the garage.

Curtis slurring, "My dad is dead, dead, Dad is dead."

Nate replies, "I know. Now, get in the car."

Curtis screams out, "Ok, but let's go to KFC."

The car lights glare off the counter top as I walk in, and say, "Mom, stop cleaning. All day you have been cleaning, now stop."

Kate, Mom, and I sit in the reconstructed room, but I can't see the difference. The table is still there, just a bit more wood showing is all; there are indents in the carpet from the bed's feet.

Soon, they're off to sleep and I am left to deal with the shadow of The Scene and the doorbell light.

Day 49

Kate walks out, "You look like you just saw a ghost."

I reply, "All fuckin' night."

"What do you mean?"

"I don't know, maybe I was scared, maybe I saw him, but I'm pretty sure he is still here. I couldn't stop seeing his face in that damn chair."

Mom walks out and says, "Oh Molly, you are just seeing things, he is gone."

"I sure hope so."

*

I open the door and get in the car. It hits my eyes like the brightest light. Its light blue hue infuriates me. I scream, "Oh my God, Mom, seriously? You really are crazy."

Kate asks, "What?"

"Look up there, on that box, far away from the garbage can I threw it in," I point to the plastic object wrapped in its black cord.

"Tweets, what is wrong with you? It is broken, come

on," Kate says.

Mom can only laugh, for she has no excuse this time.

Soon we are all laughing, Mom cries, "Please, Molly, stop, you are going to make me pee my pants."

I haven't been to church in years, but Mom wanted to go tonight, for the Good Friday service. We walk in the door, and I see and smell my childhood. We slide into a row in the back; the hard wooden pew forces my body upright. Organ pipes blare, and everyone stands and turns around. I lag behind, but get up and turn. My eyes lock on the huge cross Pastor carries down the aisle in a slow, dignified stride. He is wearing a black robe, followed by two boys in robes with smaller crosses and smaller strides. They approach the altar and carefully place the crosses in holders. The two boys light candles, as Pastor approaches the podium.

I don't recall such a theatrical tradition.

Pastor's words capture my thoughts as he says, "This Friday we call *good* is a time of somber reflection, as we are attentive to the mystery of the cross. The fact is, we are celebrating his death only because from that death flows forgiveness and life."

His words quickly fade out —the church, Mom, Kate, Dad, it's overwhelming.

Pastor calls, "Please stand as we sing hymn 447."

Kate and I look to each other for an answer, but there isn't one.

The organ takes over as I close my eyes and focus on darkness, but only light shines through me.

*

I'm on the last line of the eulogy when I awake from the days of his death. The present is the coffin in front of me. I'm finished reading, and I approach the rectangle of timber that holds him. I read it without a tear. I sit back down between Mom and Kate, as Pastor continues the service. His words echo, "Now, please take out your hymnal and we will sing hymn 447."

I grab my hymnal and search for the *hymn of the week*.

We are at the casket for the final time. I lean in for the last kiss, the last sight of him. The funeral lady drops the lid and his face melts from my eyes. We follow the crate as she wheels it out of the chapel. Down the tunnel of people I see the hearse backed up to the door. This was the door we always entered in. There are many doors to the building, but when we came to church, Dad always parked on this side.

My steps are deliberate and even as I follow the box. I can see the end of the ropes. The crowd is not smiling. Victory is mourned, but only today. This is the last ritual, as we parade his bones to flames. Cremation will be the end. Only ashes will remain, but the burning will only evaporate the frame. The creation it cradles is now content, in the form of true light and freshly mowed green grass.

*

Home

I awake and turn toward The Scene but it is finally gone, and today I will be too. I hurry down the stairs to get ready. Half-way down, I take the jump of my youth. I'm in the air and I'm free. My feet land hard on the basement floor, and I recognize the strength of my future.

I'm packing my bag, and taking in the pictures on the walls. Mom calls down to me, "Come on, Molls, we got to get to the airport."

I head back upstairs. Standing in the kitchen, my smile is huge. I would give anything for him to be here. I don't know why, but I want it back. Kate and Mom are in the car, but I'm still stuck here. Finally, my legs move, but tears fill my eyes. I breathe in the house, my childhood home.

"Goodbye, Dad, goodbye."

*

Alone, I sit waiting to board the plane that takes me back to my life. As people walk by, I close my eyes and envision an earlier moment.

I am standing with my teammates on the first tee box, as Dad drives up in his cart with Jackson, "Hey Skeets, we are going to go ahead of you."

A horn startles me and my eyes pop open. It's the typical airport scene. There is an electric cart coming my way, driven by an airport employee with travelers on seats, and a flatbed on the back. The light flashes and the horn blares, warning all to get out of the way. As it goes by, I notice, like I always do, big black numbers label it car number 47. My eyes close, and I fall back into my vision.

Dad hits his tee shot right down the middle. "When you coming home, Skeets?"

"I'm not sure, Dad. I may be a while. I gotta' practice. But keep the garage door open for me."

"It'll be open when you get home, Skeets. Oh, and Skeets – "

"Yeah, Dad."

He hops back into his cart, "Hit 'em straight, Skeets, you don't want to get stuck in the trees."

####

Made in the USA
Las Vegas, NV
17 December 2023